© **Copyright 2020 - All rights reserved.**

The content contained within this book may not be reproduced, duplicated or transmitted without direct written permission from the author or the publisher.

Under no circumstances will any blame or legal responsibility be held against the publisher, or author, for any damages, reparation, or monetary loss due to the information contained within this book, either directly or indirectly.

Legal Notice:
This book is copyright protected. It is only for personal use. You cannot amend, distribute, sell, use, quote or paraphrase any part, or the content within this book, without the consent of the author or publisher.

Disclaimer Notice:
Please note the information contained within this document is for educational and entertainment purposes only. All effort has been executed to present accurate, up to date, reliable, complete information. No warranties of any kind are declared or implied. Readers acknowledge that the author is not engaged in the rendering of legal, financial, medical or professional advice. The content within this book has been derived from various sources. Please consult a licensed professional before attempting any techniques outlined in this book.

By reading this document, the reader agrees that under no circumstances is the author responsible for any losses, direct or indirect, that are incurred as a result of the use of the information contained within this document, including, but not limited to, errors, omissions, or inaccuracies.

The LOW-FODMAP

DIET COOKBOOK

101 recipes for your low-FODMAP diet & for relief IBS and Other Digestive Disorders

28 DAY HELPFUL MEAL PLANS

ROBERT DICKENS & ANITA ROSE

Table of Contents

Introduction 9

The Low-FODMAP Basics 10

   1: The Low-FODMAP Principles 10
      Stacking 12
      Fermentation 12
   2: How Food Can Cause Digestive Problems 13
   3: Prebiotics and Probiotics 14
   4: Irritable Bowel Syndrome (IBS) and How to Relieve It ... 15
   5: The Benefits of a Low-FODMAP Diet 17
   6: Low-FODMAP Food Guide 18
      Foods with low-FODMAP 20
      Foods with Higt-FODM 22
   Frequently Asked Questions 24

28-Day Meal Plan 28
      Week 1 30
      Week 2 32
      Week 3 34
      Week 4 36
      Staple ingredients 38

Measurement conversions 40

Breakfast 43
   Egg Wraps `VEGETARIAN` 44
   Basil Omelet with Smashed Tomato `VEGETARIAN` 45
   Tomato Omelet `VEGETARIAN` 46
   Banana Porridge `VEGAN` 47
   Breakfast Wrap `VEGETARIAN` 48
   Scrambled Tofu `VEGAN` 49
   Peanut Butter Bowl `VEGETARIAN` 50
   Quinoa Porridge `VEGAN` 51
   Banana Oatcakes `VEGETARIAN` 52
   French Toast Casserole `VEGAN` 53
   Rhubarb Ginger Granola Bowl `VEGETARIAN` 54
   Crepes and Berries `VEGETARIAN` 55

Carrot Cake Porridge `VEGAN` 56
Summer Berry Smoothie `VEGETARIAN` 57
Mixed Berry & Yogurt Granola Bar `VEGETARIAN` 58
Breakfast Tortillas `VEGETARIAN` 59
Green Smoothie `VEGETARIAN` 60

Lunch 63

Carrot and Walnut Salad `VEGAN` 64
Tomato and Green Bean Salad `VEGETARIAN` 65
Corn Salad `VEGAN` 66
Ham Salad 67
Basil Vinaigrette Salad Dressing `VEGAN` 68
Thai Pumpkin Noodle Soup `VEGAN` 69
Pesto Noodles `VEGETARIAN` 70
Hawaiian Toasted Sandwich 71
Chicken Wrap 72
Pesto Toasted Sandwich 73
Quiche in Ham Cups 74
Savory Muffins `VEGETARIAN` 75
Feta, Chicken, and Pepper Sandwich 76
Rice & Zucchini Slice `VEGETARIAN` 77
Cranberry Chocolate Chip Energy Bites `VEGAN` 78
Cucumber salad `VEGETARIAN` 79
Cheese, Ham, and Spinach Muffins 80

Dinner 83

Cheesy Chicken 84
Pork Tacos with Pineapple Salsa 85
Coconut Crusted Fish 86
Bolognese 88
Minestrone 89
Frittata `VEGETARIAN` 90
Tofu Skewers `VEGAN` 92
Baked Chicken Alfredo 94
Burgers 96
Day-Before Lamb Stew 98
Vegetable Fried Rice `VEGETARIAN` 99
Tuna, Bacon Quinoa Bowl 100
Roasted Pumpkin and Carrot Soup `VEGAN` 101
Feta Meatball 102

Spicy Tacos 103
Gnocchi **VEGETARIAN** 104
Vegan Curry **VEGAN** 106

Side Dishes and Starters 108

Parmesan Mayo Corn on the Cob **VEGETARIAN** 110
Garden Medley **VEGAN** 111
Zucchini Fritters **VEGETARIAN** 112
Pumpkin Cornbread **VEGETARIAN** 113
Veggie Dip **VEGETARIAN** 114
Mashed Potatoes **VEGETARIAN** 115
Festive Stuffing **VEGAN** 116
Chicken Cheese Fritters 117
Rice Paper "Spring Rolls" with Satay Sauce **VEGAN** 118
Chive Dip **VEGAN** 120
Roast Vegetables **VEGAN** 121
Beetroot Dip **VEGAN** 122

Drinks 125

Strawberry Basil Soda **VEGAN** 126
Raspberry Mocktail **VEGAN** 127
Electrolyte Refresher **VEGETARIAN** 128
Strawberry Lemonade **VEGAN** 129
Cranberry Lemonade **VEGAN** 130
Mock Piña Colada **VEGAN** 131
Hot Ginger and Lemon **VEGAN** 132
Spiced Hot Chocolate **VEGAN** 133
Cinnamon and Cranberry Fizz **VEGAN** 134
Golden Coffee **VEGETARIAN** 135
White Matcha Latte **VEGAN** 136
Hot Oat Milk **VEGAN** 137
Fruity Mimosa **VEGAN** 138

Smoothies 141

Basic Smoothie Base 142
Smoothie Bowl **VEGAN** 144
Kale, Ginger, and Pineapple Smoothie **VEGAN** 145
Strawberry Smoothie **VEGAN** 146
Blueberry, Lime, and Coconut Smoothie **VEGAN** 147
Pineapple, Strawberry, Raspberry Smoothie **VEGAN** 148

Tropical Smoothie `VEGAN` 149
Green Smoothie `VEGAN` 150
Blueberry Lime Smoothie `VEGETARIAN` 151
Blueberry, Kiwi, and Mint `VEGETARIAN` 152
Fruit Salad Smoothie `VEGETARIAN` 153
Protein Smoothie `VEGAN` 154
Cranberry Almond Bowl `VEGETARIAN` 155

Snacks 157
Sweet and Savory Popcorn `VEGAN` 158
Quinoa Muffins `VEGETARIAN` 159
Lemon Coconut Cupcakes `VEGETARIAN` 160
Chocolate Peanut Butter Energy Bites `VEGAN` 161
Blueberry Muffins `VEGAN` 162
Summer Popsicle `VEGAN` 163
Pineapple, Yogurt on Rice Cakes `VEGETARIAN` 164
Salted Caramel Pumpkin Seeds `VEGETARIAN` 165
Orange Biscuits `VEGETARIAN` 166
Coconut Bites `VEGETARIAN` 167
Carrot Parsnip Chips `VEGAN` 168
Baked Oat Cup `VEGETARIAN` 169
Energy Bars `VEGETARIAN` 170

Sweet Treats 173
Chia Pudding `VEGAN` 174
Berry Crumble `VEGETARIAN` 175
Banana Birthday Cake with Lemon Icing `VEGETARIAN` 176
Brownie Cupcakes with Vanilla Icing `VEGETARIAN` 178
Rhubarb Custard Cup `VEGETARIAN` 180
Fluffy Pancakes `VEGETARIAN` 181
Chocolate Fudge Sauce `VEGAN` 182
Chocolate Raspberry Dessert `VEGETARIAN` 183
Christmas Mince Pie `VEGETARIAN` 184
Strawberry Ice Cream `VEGAN` 186
Ginger Cookies `VEGAN` 187
PB&J Mug Cake `VEGETARIAN` 188
Lemon Bar `VEGETARIAN` 189

Introduction

Many people around the world struggle with digestion problems. These issues can cause a wide variety of symptoms that can be frustrating and disrupt daily life. While some symptoms can be treated using medication, there are some that cannot. For many people, lifestyle changes are the main ways that the digestive system will start to function in a healthy manner. Lifestyle changes can be made in various areas including changing sleep habits, stress levels, the environment around us, and our diet.

For individuals who spend every day trying to cope with digestive issues, life can become frustrating. Many of these individuals will see their symptoms increase when they eat certain foods. If the symptoms become unmanageable, every day becomes a fight. This often includes dealing with pain that is unbearable. The pain related to digestive issues should be addressed with the help of a healthcare professional who will often suggest that the best option for the individual is to start restricting the foods that they eat.

This book is designed to help those individuals with digestive issues who are just beginning to learn how to cook digestion-friendly food. The diet that will be focused on is the low-FODMAP diet. As a book, the following is aimed at individuals who are looking to start eating healthier. It also aims to guide people struggling with digestive issues, those who are not good at cooking, as well as people who are new to cooking.

As a guide, this book will provide information about the principles of a low-FODMAP diet. These include aspects of the diet, how it is helpful, and the steps involved in implementing the diet. There will also be information on how different foods can affect the body, with a specific look at the digestive system and the way it functions. Digestive issues related to food can be frustrating, and the most common digestive struggle experienced is irritable bowel syndrome (IBS). This book will look at both IBS, specifically, and digestive struggles, in general, to see how the low-FODMAP diet can put someone on the path to a healthier life with less digestive difficulties.

The guide will not only increase knowledge about the positives of a low-FODMAP diet and how it can improve digestion, but it will also provide a list of foods that can and cannot be eaten on the diet due to the interaction they have with our body. Once the basic knowledge is understood, there will be a more in-depth look at what goes into this diet.

A 28-day meal plan with a shopping list is also included in the book. Menu planning will be explained with examples of how to best go about the process. Lastly, there are over 100 easy, budget-friendly recipes that will kick-start the journey to healthier eating.

The Low-FODMAP Basics

There are different ways to set yourself up to successfully implement a healthy lifestyle. The first step is to understand what makes up a lifestyle. Many people think that if they exercise, they will be healthy, but this is not the only factor when it comes to living a healthy lifestyle. A healthy life is comprised of habits created in several areas including diet, exercise, mental health, and the environment.

The following section will discuss the basics of a low-FODMAP diet, along with the basic principles, benefits, and best foods to eat. There will also be information on one of the most common digestive issues IBS and how certain foods can cause digestive issues.

1: The Low-FODMAP Principles

As a diet, low-FODMAP aims to improve digestion and digestion-related issues. FODMAP refers to carbohydrates, a form of sugar that is found in foods and is used for energy.

FODMAP stands for Fermentable, Oligosaccharides, Disaccharides, Monosaccharides, and Polyols; these are simply the scientific terms for the various carbohydrates that draw water into the intestines and can then cause digestive symptoms. These carbohydrates can be found in a number of different foods, and some foods contain one type, while others may have numerous ones. FODMAP foods are the only types of food that ferment in the digestive system. Some symptoms that are caused by FODMAP foods include gas, bloating, nausea, abdominal pain, constipation, and an upset stomach. The foods that are listed in the "do not eat" category are not unhealthy but are often the cause of digestive issues.

For individuals who struggle with digestive issues or other disorders, this diet gives the body a chance to heal the problems in the digestive system by eliminating foods that cause those problems. The aim of this diet is to discover which foods that fall under the FODMAP guidelines the body can tolerate. This is done in a controlled manner, usually with the assistance of a dietician. Through a specific program, the trigger symptoms can be reduced and a nutritional balance of foods can be determined. The diet is broken down into stages for the best results.

- **Stage 1 - Restriction/elimination:** This stage can take between two to eight weeks. During this time, food is strictly chosen to avoid high-FODMAP foods. By doing this, the triggers found in high-FODMAP foods are reduced and any symptoms related to IBS or other digestive issues will be reduced or completely relieved. It is important to be strict during this stage since it is time for your body to discover what "normal" is. It also allows the body to reset. This time can also be used to see what other triggers you might have in your life. These can be stress, poor sleep, and other health issues.

  The next stage occurs once symptoms in the digestive system are mostly relieved.

- **Stage 2 - Re-challenge:** When moving into this stage, it is time to start adding high-FODMAP foods back into the diet slowly. This process helps determine which foods irritate the digestive system. The restriction is still in place, but one test food from one of the high-FODMAP categories is added into your diet for a short period of time to see which categories act as triggers.

  When reintroducing a FODMAP group, it is best to select a food that has one FODMAP. This food should be eaten in increasingly larger amounts over a period of a few days. By slowly increasing the quantity of the food, you are testing it to see what symptoms will be triggered and how severe they will be. It is a recommendation that only one food per category be tested at a time since it can be difficult to know which FODMAP is causing symptoms if there is more than one present. In general, one food should be tested each week, and if you have no reaction, then you can completely reintroduce it once you have finished testing the other FODMAPs. If you have a strong reaction, then you can consider reintroducing it in smaller amounts or eliminating it completely.
  Between groups, there needs to be a time frame for the body to reset back to complete elimination, which allows any symptoms experienced to settle down. This should typically be about three days.

  With foods that do not irritate the system as much, the purpose is to discover the level of tolerance. It is crucial to not stay on the elimination part of the diet for a long period of time as it can cause damage to the natural bacteria in the digestive system.

- **Stage 3 - Reintroduction:** This stage is a continuation of Stage 2. During this stage, you put food back into your long-term diet. Unlike the second stage, in this one, there is no need to go back to the elimination stage. Once a food has been added back into your diet, it can stay part of your list of foods to eat, as long as it does not cause any symptoms.

- **Stage 4 - Personalization/maintenance:** After the completion of the previous stages, it is time to create a personalized tolerance food list. The foods that were determined to be intolerable will still be restricted, while others will be modified as necessary. Maintenance is done as time goes by. If a food on the list starts to cause symptoms, it is time to reevaluate it. Other factors in life may cause your tolerance or threshold, explained later in this part, to change. Changes in sleep or stress are two factors that can influence symptoms.

It is important to note that these stages will take place with a long-term eating plan in mind. This diet should not be used as a purely health-related diet, and it is not a cure for IBS and other symptoms. It should not be maintained over a long period of time with extreme restriction. Another important factor to note is that this diet takes time. It may be helpful to keep a food journal because it may aid in the elimination and reintroduction process.

Stacking

Another concept that falls under FODMAPs is stacking. This relates to the tolerance and threshold that each person has for the different FODMAPs. A threshold is determined by the symptoms experienced after a certain amount of FODMAPs is consumed. It is determined in the reintroduction phase of the diet.

Tolerance is determined by the number of foods from one FODMAP group that can be eaten. Tolerance can change over time and can relate to the portion sizes.

Stacking is related to how FODMAPs are eaten. In simple terms, when two or more servings consisting of the same FODMAPs are eaten in a close time frame, it is considered stacking. Each person has a certain amount of space in their system that can store FODMAPs. If there is no more space, symptoms will show.

Stacking occurs when the food items are from the high-FODMAP categories. Even when the foods are reintroduced and can be tolerated, when your body reaches its limit, symptoms will show. To avoid FODMAP stacking, it is best to try to mix and match foods from the low-FODMAP list. One main tip for stacking is to try to create space between meals. By leaving time between meals, the body has time to process the previous meal, and this, in turn, makes it easier for the next meal to go through your system.

Fermentation

Fermentation is a large part of FODMAPs and is involved in the digestive process. Basically, fermentation is when microorganisms such as bacteria turn carbohydrates into alcohol or lactic acid. This process usually happens in a space with no oxygen.

There are two main forms of fermentation. The first type is alcoholic, and this is typically when yeast breaks down sugars into carbon dioxide and ethanol. This is mostly used to make beer, wine, and other alcoholic drinks. The second is lactic acid fermentation. This is the breakdown of carbohydrates into lactic acid, most commonly used to make yogurt, cheese, or pickled ingredients. These two types of fermentation can happen at the same time.

Fermentation and fermented foods can be used for a wide variety of things including food preservation and the breakdown of foods that are hard to digest. Certain fermented foods also add probiotics to your system. Another benefit of fermented foods is the lowering of FODMAPs in certain foods, which allows these foods to be eaten in small amounts.

Some people believe that because fermentation breaks down carbohydrates, the FODMAPs will be lowered if the food is fermented. This is not true all the time. Some foods will have more FODMAPs after being fermented, while others will have less. Some foods are not affected by fermentation at all.

2: How Food Can Cause Digestive Problems

Digestion is the process through which the body breaks down food so that the nutrients can be absorbed. These nutrients are vital for the functioning of the body. Certain food products provide necessary nutrients, while others cause issues. Eating an unbalanced diet can lead to a lack of available nutrients for the body to absorb, which, in turn, causes cells to malfunction or die (Chi, 2019). Digestive functioning is a crucial part of the quality of life for individuals around the world.

The main section of the digestive tract where symptoms can pop up is the large intestine. The large intestine is divided into four main parts (including the colon and rectum) that absorb different nutrients. Food that the body cannot digest also passes through the large intestine (Zimmermann, 2016). A low fiber diet, traveling, stress, and eating too much dairy can all cause digestive issues.

This process of digestion is a natural one; however, some individuals will find that certain foods create issues during the process. Most foods contain nutrients that the body needs; however, those that do not contain useful nutrients create uncomfortable symptoms.

Certain digestive issues are chronic, and they are often difficult to diagnose and treat. The struggle with digestive symptoms is their link to the food that people eat on a daily basis. Eating the wrong foods can create issues such as pain, bloating, diarrhea, constipation, and other symptoms. At the same time, eating the right foods or eliminating problematic foods can reduce symptoms. When digestive symptoms are particularly bad, there are cleanses and specific diets, such as the low-FODMAP diet, that will improve the quality of life.

One question that often comes up when discussing diets is the affect alcohol has on digestion. Alcoholic drinks have some of the specific carbohydrates that are on the high-FODMAP list and are related to the slowing down of the digestive processes. However, it is not just the alcohol alone that can trigger IBS and other related symptoms. A large part of this has to do with the habits of the individual who experiences the symptoms. One of the main factors that affects these individuals is the amount of alcohol they drink; binge drinkers show a higher level of digestive symptoms. When choosing to partake in the modern culture of alcohol consumption, it is important to understand the limits of your body so that you don't consume too much alcohol and provoke digestion symptoms.

Wheat is a large contributor to FODMAPs; this is due to the high quantity of wheat products that are consumed in Western diets. At nearly every meal, there is some form of wheat product that is eaten. A simple switch away from products that contain wheat can make a big difference to digestive health.

One of the most concentrated sources of FODMAPs is garlic, which is unfortunate since garlic is one of the most common ingredients for flavoring food because of its ability to bring out the natural flavors of certain food products. The main FODMAP found in garlic is called fructan; the quantity depends on the type of garlic. While garlic is high in FODMAPS, there are many health benefits. For this reason, it should only be restricted long-term for people who have a severe sensitivity to high-FODMAP foods.

Fructose is a FODMAP that is found in all fruits. However, not all fruit is considered to be high-FODMAP due to the levels of fructose in different fruits. Fruits that are considered to be low-FODMAP are high in glucose, which is a type of sugar that does not fall into the high-FODMAP list. It must be noted that while glucose does not have an effect like fructose, it can, in high quantities, cause digestive symptoms.

Looking at vegetables, there are many that are considered high-FODMAPs. This is due to a number of factors, one of the main ones being that many vegetables contain more than one type of FODMAP. One of these is asparagus, which contains fructans, fructose, and vegetable-specific mannitol. Vegetables are an essential part of a balanced and healthy diet. Due to this, it is best to switch high-FODMAPs out of your diet and replace them with low-FODMAP vegetables such as kale, tomatoes, and carrots.

Legumes are types of beans that have a reputation for causing specific digestive symptoms, mainly gas and bloating. In the case of many legumes, the high-FODMAP qualities are directly affected by the way they are prepared. However, even when these are prepared in a way that reduces the FODMAPs, they are best consumed in extremely small qualities.

Lactose is the main FODMAP source found in dairy products. While cheese is one type of dairy that contains little to no lactose, there are certain cheeses that contain garlic and onions, making them unsuitable for this particular diet. There are a number of dairy products that are low in lactose or are even lactose-free.

There are many foods that are high in FODMAPs. However, the majority of people are not sensitive to these. Those that are not sensitive should not restrict these foods from their diet. For those who do struggle with digestive symptoms, it will be helpful to create restrictions on what FODMAPs they eat and the quantities they consume.

3: Prebiotics and Probiotics

Each person has a mixture of different bacteria that live inside their digestive system. These create what is known as an individual's "microbiome" or "microbiota." In these systems, probiotics and prebiotics can be used to help with digestive symptoms.

Probiotics are microorganisms that can improve health if the correct amount is taken. They can be found in some foods (such as fermented foods) and supplements. Some probiotics have been proven to help with abdominal pain from IBS.

Probiotics are considered to be good bacteria that can change the ecosystem in your digestive system temporarily. This includes changing the pH balance, creating unsuitable conditions for bad bacteria, and triggering the immune system to fight off certain bacteria. When taken with food, probiotic supplements can help the body produce extra vitamins. Some of the supplements even take the good bacteria directly to your large intestine for maximum effects.

Prebiotics, on the other hand, are compounds that the body cannot digest. These have a positive impact on the microbiome. They are directly supplied from your diet and are found in carbohydrates containing fructans—like garlic or onions—or in beans, nuts, and seeds. While prebiotics can be good, they can also act negatively in the digestive symptoms of people who struggle with IBS. Due to the fermentable nature of prebiotics, they can act like a super-food to the bacteria in your system. They act as a double-edged sword by increasing good bacteria but causing a reaction in even the low-FODMAP foods. This causes a chain reaction in the form of IBS symptoms. Even with the negative side of prebiotics, it is not healthy for them to be eliminated from your system. When prebiotics are removed over a period of time, the good bacteria in your system will start to die, which can be a permanent effect. The lowering of prebiotic levels is one of the main reasons that a low-FODMAP diet cannot be permanent.

Both probiotics and prebiotics are essential to your digestive health. Although prebiotics have highly fermentable qualities, they are important to the production of good bacteria. Probiotics are also part of creating a positive environment in the digestive system. A healthy digestive system is one of the key factors in helping relieve IBS symptoms.

4: Irritable Bowel Syndrome (IBS) and How to Relieve It

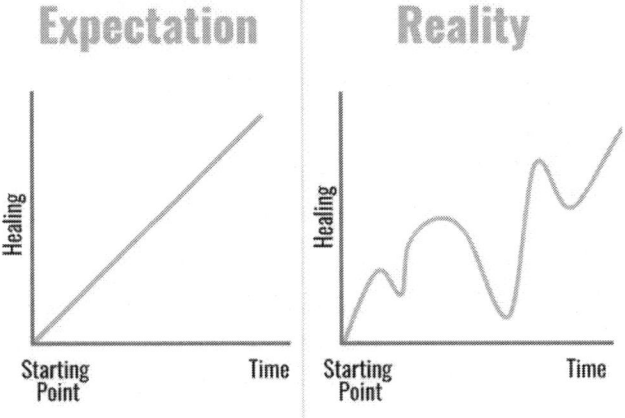

There are many disorders that can affect the digestive system; often, they are caused by the bacteria that aid in digestion. One of the most common digestive disorders is IBS. When an individual suffers from this disorder, they experience symptoms that range from abdominal pain to constipation to diarrhea. The basic description describes IBS as an impairment of the intestinal functioning. This malfunctioning can create struggles in the individual's day-to-day functioning; this can lead to avoiding social interactions and taking days off work.

In a digestive system that is functioning normally, the intestines contract during the process. For those who struggle with IBS, the intestine contractions are uncoordinated, with some lasting longer or shorter than usual. These uncoordinated contractions can cause a large amount of abdominal pain and irregular bowel movements. External conditions that can also cause symptoms of IBS are stress or a hormone imbalance. While the underlying cause of IBS is not known, triggers can be linked strongly to diet or food allergies, such as dairy or gluten allergies (Angelle, 2017). It should be noted that each person will experience symptoms differently.

Certain foods also make the gut uncomfortable and cause IBS symptoms. This is because of the impact the food has on the bacteria in our gut. For example, eating foods that are high in calories, sugar, and fat can cause harmful bacteria in our guts to grow faster than normal. Feeding those bad bacteria can cause them to overtake the good, healthy bacteria, which leads to discomfort and IBS symptoms.

One of the major symptoms experienced with IBS is abdominal pain. The abdomen is the space between your ribs and the top of your hips. The type of pain experienced can vary from sharp to stabbing to cramping to pressure. This pain is linked to the nervous system. Certain FODMAPs pull water into the intestines, which, in turn, creates a build-up of gas and leads to the abdomen muscles spasming and causing pain. The nervous system cannot tell where the pain in your abdomen is coming from specifically, so your brain relays a message of pain that is spread out across your abdomen.

Constipation also causes gas to build up and your intestines to swell. When there is too much swelling, the stretched intestines create pain. In this case, the brain can tell the exact point the pain is coming from. With the brain receiving pain messages from multiple places in the abdomen, there will be pain in every section of the digestive system. It must never be assumed that the pain is IBS-related without a diagnosis since there are other reasons for abdominal pain.

After the abdomen comes the pelvic floor. Basically, the pelvic floor is what supports your organs. This floor is made of muscles, tendons, and ligaments that are attached to the bones that make up your pelvis. One of the functions of the pelvic floor is to control the muscles that are related to using the bathroom. It also resists internal pressure so that we have control over our bladder when we laugh or cough. When dysfunctions and issues arise, they can cause pain to spread outside of the abdomen. Without the help of the pelvic floor, those who struggle with IBS will experience a greater struggle.

For women who struggle with IBS, it is common for the symptoms to worsen when they are menstruating. There are a number of hormones that are produced and released during this cycle, and they all serve different purposes. One hormone is progesterone, which acts as a natural muscle relaxant. With the abdominal muscles relaxed, it can be more difficult to go to the bathroom. However, once the progesterone levels drop, the opposite is likely to happen. As these levels drop, there is a release of what is known as prostaglandins. These are what cause contractions to start; unfortunately, they do not stay in the uterus and spread through the body causing pain in various places, including the intestines. The drop in hormones can also cause bloating, which then creates more intense symptoms.

There is no cure for IBS, but there are ways to manage the symptoms. Some professionals will prescribe medication, usually a probiotic. One of the main ways to control the symptoms is a change in diet. The low-FODMAP diet is often encouraged since it allows the individual to determine the specific foods that cause a flare-up of symptoms. After determining that, the person can remove those foods and stick to a healthy lifestyle to prevent more flare-ups.

In many cases, people have reported positive effects that a low-FODMAP diet has had on their IBS symptoms. The majority of those who reported back to professionals showed improvements in more than one symptom. Three of the main reductions were seen in bloating, abdominal pain, and gas. These reductions could be a result of the probiotic effect that certain foods have when digested.

If you are planning on seeing a professional to discuss whether you have IBS or not, there are a few questions that you should be prepared to ask. First, you should determine if you will need to have a colonoscopy. Some symptoms are a normal part of IBS or digestive issues, while others aren't and may raise red flags that should be checked out immediately.

Women who are experiencing IBS should check with their doctor to determine if they should see a gynecologist. This second opinion is needed for some women as the female anatomy is extremely complicated. There are a number of other health issues that have symptoms similar to IBS.

How will you be able to tell the difference between IBS and other health issues? With IBS, it is important to know what symptoms to look out for. If you are experiencing symptoms that you are not used to experiencing, it is important that you see your doctor. A professional will help you to know what symptoms you experience are from IBS so that you can be vigilant.

5: The Benefits of a Low-FODMAP Diet

A low-FODMAP diet can benefit individuals in a number of ways. One of the main benefits is the effect on digestion, especially for those who suffer from specific disorders that impact digestion. Those on the diet often experience less gas, bloating, and abdominal pain. Relief from these symptoms leads to a number of other benefits.

When bloating decreases, there is a physical difference, and individuals will feel their clothes fit better and confidence will increase. With a decrease in constipation and diarrhea, there will be less stress when going into social situations because the worry about making a run to the bathroom is minimal. This decrease in stress will have a positive effect in everyday life, from mood to improvements in the workplace to better relationships (Paul, 2017).

Food is used to fuel our bodies. With every bite taken, the body tries to break down the food into nutrients that can be used. For these nutrients to be absorbed, the body has to use enzymes to break them down small enough to enter the bloodstream. Enzymes are what are known as catalysts. Catalysts help start changes or speed up slow changes. During digestion, enzymes break down the bonds between molecules. Each enzyme is unique and breaks down one type of compound. An example of this is the enzyme galactose, which breaks down glucose. The tension put onto the compound by an enzyme causes it to break apart into parts that are small enough to enter the bloodstream.

From the moment you take your first bite of food, enzymes are working on breaking the food down; the enzymes in your saliva help in the breakdown of carbohydrates and proteins. As the food works its way through your digestive system, the different enzymes will work together to break down the nutrients that are needed by the body. Enzymes are a natural part of the digestive system and have many benefits. There are not many man-made enzymes that can be bought. This is why certain foods are beneficial when included in a diet.

As a whole, the low-FODMAP diet has many benefits. These extend to every area of an individual's life. By following the diet, uncomfortable digestion symptoms can be minimized or eliminated and healthy functioning can be restored. This leads to a healthier life.

While there are benefits to a low-FODMAP diet, as with any diet, there are a few risks. The major one is nutritional deficiency, but there are other concerns. One of the biggest risks is the inappropriate use of the diet. There are some who will use the diet to diagnose gluten sensitivity when there are no digestive symptoms present.

When planning to start this diet, it is recommended to work with a healthcare professional, specifically a dietician, since not everyone will respond well to food restrictions. This is especially crucial for those with food allergies or restrictions due to health conditions. Some changes in the low-FODMAP diet may not mix well with allergies or dietary restrictions, and a dietician or medical professional can assist with accommodating these requirements.

tarting any diet comes with challenges that need to be worked out. One challenge is to not start changing everything in one swoop. If you are on medications or supplements, it is not ideal to start changing everything at the same time. Doing this can cause negative reactions and lead to more serious symptoms. Working with professionals gives your body the best chance of having a positive reaction to the changes being made.

Many people become frustrated and stop a diet because they are not seeing any immediate results. It is never good to start a change such as a diet with the expectation of seeing improvements after a day or two, and the low-FODMAP diet is no exception. While there are some who will feel changes sooner, those who do not may get frustrated and give up too soon.

When starting this diet with the goal of reducing IBS symptoms, it is important to set boundaries. Not everyone around you will understand the struggle you face with IBS and its symptoms. This is where boundaries are important as they will aid in the success of the diet. The benefits of eating a low-FODMAP diet will be for nothing if others are able to walk in and destroy all your progress. Other people will probably need time to process and respond when you tell them about your struggle because they may not understand why you are cutting different food items from your diet.

You also need to set boundaries for yourself; to benefit fully from this diet, you cannot let people dictate what you can or cannot eat. Do not be afraid to ask people around you for help and support. By talking to others and ensuring those you live with do not feel deprived of any food they enjoy, you will ensure that you not only reap the benefits of eating low-FODMAP but that those around you do too.

6: Low-FODMAP Food Guide

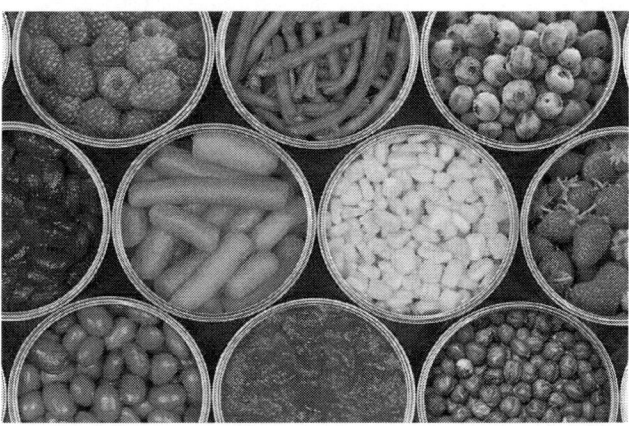

Later in this section, you will see a list of the low-FODMAP foods that can be eaten and the high-FODMAP foods that should be restricted and reintroduced to determine tolerance levels. Before we get to that, we need to look at some specifics related to dieting.

Words that are often used in eating plans and diets are portion sizes and serving sizes. Broadly speaking, portion size is the amount you choose to eat. It must be noted that portion size is not the same as a serving size.

In the FODMAP diet, the term serving size is used frequently. Serving sizes can be seen on food labels; this is the producer's recommendation of how much of an ingredient should be used. Serving sizes can also be found on recipes and websites that give recommendations according to specific diets. However, due to the number of variations in suggested serving sizes, it will be up to each person to find a balance in what serving sizes work. While serving sizes are specific to the individual, it is important when doing the low-FODMAP diet that the individual understands how FODMAPs affect digestion. This is important because it will help an individual know which foods should be consumed in smaller servings.

Restricting certain foods from your diet will cause an imbalance in the nutrients in the body. Nutrients are compounds that are found in foods, and they are essential for functioning. There are two umbrella categories that nutrients fall under: macronutrients and micronutrients.

Macronutrients are found in carbohydrates, fats, and proteins. These make up a large part of an individual's daily diet and provide the body with energy. Micronutrients are chemicals that the body needs for growth. Many foods today are lacking in nutrients; these nutrients are replaced with excess energy. This is due to the body's natural process, which converts carbohydrates into sugars. These sugars are then stored as fat if the body does not use these nutrients.

Nutrients that are in danger of becoming too low on this diet are fiber, vitamins, and protein. Fiber will be limited when eating low-FODMAPs because it is mainly found in fruits, vegetables, and grains that have high-FODMAPs. However, there are many small ways to ensure that fiber is included in the meals. Some ways include adding flaxseeds or replacement powders found in health stores.

Vitamin D and calcium are vitamins that suffer when starting out on this diet. This is due to the restrictions on dairy, which is the main source of these nutrients. There are ways to increase these nutrients, such as adding in foods like fatty fish, leafy green vegetables, and supplements.

Protein is mainly a concern for those who are choosing to follow the diet as a vegan or vegetarian. While there are other sources of protein in legumes, dairy, and nuts, it can be difficult to get a sufficient amount of nutrients into the body. The best way to have a sufficient amount of protein is a combination of meat, legumes, dairy, and nuts.

Onions and garlic are used as the main forms of flavoring in Western diets; however, on the low-FODMAP diet, these fall into the high-FODMAP category. On the positive side, this diet will teach you how to flavor food in different ways that are just as tasty and delicious as food cooked with onions and garlic.

To be able to better understand how to flavor your food, it is important to keep a supply of herbs around. You should also take into account that some herbs and spices will keep their flavor better if they are fresh, while others will keep their flavor when dried. If you want to achieve a certain flavor, then it is in your own interest to look at what substitutes can be made that will get a flavor closest to what you want. For example, many people will swap regular onions with the green part of leeks or spring onions.

Now that we've looked at the ideas behind the low-FODMAP diet, here are the foods that should and should not be consumed.

Foods with low-FODMAP

VEGETABLES

- AROMATIC HERB (all)
- AUBERGINES
- BAMBOO SHOOTS
- BOK CHOY
- BROCCOLI
- BUTTERNUT SQUASH
- CARROTS
- CELERY
- CHARD
- CORN COB
- COURGETTE
- CUCUMBERS
- FENNEL
- GINGER
- GREEN BEANS
- KALE
- LETTUCE (all)
- NAPA CABBAGE
- OKRA
- PALMITO
- PARSNIPS
- POTATOES
- RADISHES
- RED CABBAGE
- RED PEPPERONI
- SPRING ONION (green part)
- SOY SHOOTS
- SPINACH
- SWEET POTATOES
- TOMATOES
- TURNIP
- WATER CHESTNUT

FRUITS

- BANANA (unripe)
- CANTALOUPE MELON
- **CITRUS FRUITS:** orange, clementine, lime, lemon, tangerine, grapefruit
- CRANBERRY
- COCONUT
- **FOREST FRUITS:** strawberries, raspberries, blueberries
- GRAPES
- GUAVA (ripe)
- HONEYDEW MELON
- KIWI
- LITCHI
- MARACUJÁ (passion fruit)
- PAPAYA
- PINEAPPLE
- PITAYA (dragon's fruit)
- RHUBARB

CEREALS

Cereals, pasta, bread and crackers made only with the following flours:

- AMARANTH
- BUCKWHEAT
- CORN
- MILLET
- OATS
- QUINOA
- RICE
- SORGHUM
- TAPIOCA
- TEFF

HIGH-PROTEIN FOODS

- EGGS
- ALL UNPROCESSED MEAT, POULTRY, FISH AND SEA FRUITS
- SEITAN, TEMPEH, TOFU
- SHELLED EDAMAME
- BOILED CHICKPEAS AND LENTILS
- **DRIED FRUIT AND SEEDS:** peanuts, peanut butter, Almond Butter, almonds, hazelnuts, walnuts, Brazil nuts, macadamia nuts, pecans, Pine nuts, hemp seeds, Chia seeds, sunflower seeds, flax seed, Sesame seeds, pumpkin seeds

DAIRY PRODUCT AND SUBSTITUTES

- RICE MILK
- ALMOND MILK
- **CHEESES:** brie, camembert, cheddar, Comté, emmental, feta, fontina, gorgonzola, Gruyere, parmesan, pecorino cheese, taleggio cheese
- GOAT'S CHEESE (aged)
- MILK, YOGURT AND ICE CREAM (LACTOSE-FREE)
- COCONUT YOGURT

CONDIMENTS

- BUTTER
- KETCHUP
- MARGARINE
- MAYONNAISE
- MUSTARD
- OLIVE
- SOY SAUCE

SPICES
TOMATO PASTE
VEGETABLE OIL
VINEGAR

SWEETENERS

DARK CHOCOLATE
MAPLE SYRUP

RICE SYRUP
SUGAR
ORGANIC CANE SUGAR

DRINKS

WATER
COCONUT WATER
BEER

CAFFÈ
TEA (excluding cha and oolong)
HERBAL TEAS (excluding chamomile, fennel, dandelion)
VINE (excluding sweet and fortified wines)

Foods with Higt-FODMAP

VEGETABLES
- GARLIC
- ONIONS
- APARAGUS
- **BEANS:**
- black, broad, kidney, lima, soya
- CAULIFOWER
- MANGE TOUT
- MUSHROOMS
- PEAS
- SCALLIONS
- SPRING ONIONS (white part)

FRUITS
- APPLES
- APRICOT
- AVOCADO
- BANANA (ripe)
- BLACKBERRIES
- GRAPEFRUIT
- MANGO
- PEACHES
- PEARS
- PLUMS
- RAISINS
- SULTANAS
- WATERMELON

CEREALS
- BREAD, GRAINS and PASTA
- BARLEY
- BRAN
- COUS COUS
- GNOCCHI
- GRANOLA
- MUESLI
- MUFFINS
- RYE
- SEMOLINA
- SPELT
- WHEAT FOODS (Bread, cereal, pasta)

HIGH-PROTEIN FOODS
- CHORIZO
- SAUSAGES
- PROCESSED MEAT (check ingredients)
- DRIED FRUIT AND SEEDS: Cashews, Pistachio

DAIRY PRODUCT AND SUBSTITUTES
- COW MILK
- GOAT MILK
- SHEEP'S MILK
- GOAT'S CHEESE (soft)
- SOY MILK (made with soy beans)
- MILK, YOGURT AND ICE CREAM (with lactose)
- BUTERMILK
- CREAM
- CUSTARD
- SOUR CREAM
- CREAM CHEESE
- RICOTA CHEESE

CONDIMENTS
- HOMMUS DIP
- JAM (mixed berries)
- PASTA SAUCE (cream based)
- RELISH
- TZATZIKI DIP

SWEETENERS
- AGAVE
- HIGH FRUCOSE CORN SYRUP (HFCS)
- HONEY
- INULIN
- ISOMALT
- MALTTOL
- MANNITOL
- SORBITOL
- XYLITOL

DRINKS
- APPLE JUICE
- PEAR JUICE
- MANGO JUICE
- SODAS WITH HFCS
- HERBAL TEAS (only: chamomile, fennel, dandelion)

Scan QR code to download this list

Frequently Asked Questions

I am going to have to stay on this diet forever?

A long-term restriction is definitely not the goal. The main goal of this diet is to reintroduce as many foods back into your diet as possible. The way foods are reintroduced and permanently removed will have to be decided during the process.

Why are there restrictions on onion and garlic but the infused oils are safe to use?

FODMAPs are soluble in water, but they are not in fat. When an onion is placed into a stock or broth, it will leave the FODMAPs behind in the mixture when removed. In an oil-based mixture, the flavor is left behind but the FODMAPS do not linger.

Can I have a cheat day?

This is a big no-no when it comes to this diet. When removing the high-FODMAPS, the goal is to let the body expel the high-FODMAPS so there is a clean slate to start the reintroduction process. Having even a small amount of high-FODMAPs will set you back, and the process will need to be started from scratch.

Am I going to be able to eat the foods I love again?

The main goal is to get back to the point where only the minimum food items are cut out of your diet. However, there is a large number of people who are content to avoid certain high-FODMAPs almost completely.

When will I notice improvements?

It depends on the individual. Some notice changes in 48 hours, while it can take weeks for others to notice even the smallest improvement.

Are there resources that I can use to help with my low-FODMAP journey?

Yes, if you go online, there are a number of websites that give information on the low-FODMAP diet. There are also websites that give recipes specific to this diet. One of the main ones is Monash University. They have also developed an app that shows foods that can or cannot be eaten.
https://www.monashfodmap.com/

Is there a limit to the number of low-FODMAPs I can eat?

Yes, any type of food has its limit. No matter what food you eat, there needs to be some form of boundaries. When you eat too many low-FODMAPs, it is called stacking, and it can cause a flare-up of symptoms.

Can I be sensitive to all FODMAPs?

No, some people can have a sensitivity to most of the categories of FODMAPs; however, there is a very low chance of reacting to all of them. If you are not remembering what foods you are testing, then it is time to start a diary. This will help you to keep track of the foods you test and which ones cause you to experience symptoms. Another tip for this is to make sure you are on a strict elimination and only testing one food at a time. If you are still struggling, try to adjust the amount you are eating in a sitting.

Can a food sensitivity test show me what my IBS triggers are?

No. IBS and food sensitivities or allergies are not the same things. IBS is when the food is not absorbed into your body completely. On the other hand, a food sensitivity or allergy is when your body—your immune system, to be specific—reacts negatively to food that is considered to be normal. In short, your body treats a food as if it was a virus, which causes a reaction that is an annoyance, like hives, or it can be life-threatening. The sensitivity test shows which foods cause your antibodies to react.

Why do my symptoms get worse after I exercise?

This can be due to a number of factors. One is that a high-intensity exercise routine can push your abdominal wall against your internal organs, which releases stress hormones and, in turn, causes symptoms to feel worse.

Is sugar low-FODMAP?

Some symptoms of IBS are caused by an inability to absorb fructose. Fructose, when in combination with glucose, can be absorbed. For this reason, the low-FODMAP diet aims to limit fructose. Regular brown or white sugar is made up of an even amount of fructose and glucose. For this reason, these types of sugars are low-FODMAP, although there is a limit as to how much should be eaten.

What should I do if there is blood in my stool?

Any time you see blood in your stool, the first thing you should do is call or visit a doctor. While it is not always serious, it is important to see where the blood is coming from. Google is not a doctor, so always seek medical help. There are some types of bleeding that will need emergency care. However, you should talk to your doctor and let them help you plan for what to do in a situation where there is bleeding.

Why are low-FODMAP fruits added to the high-FODMAP list when they are dried?

In the process of drying fruit, the FODMAPs in the fruit are concentrated. When the FODMAPs are concentrated, the fructose quantity increases, making it fall into the high-FODMAP list. As a rule, dried fruits should be limited to as few as possible.

Is it true that sourdough bread is tolerated better than other bread?

Due to the fermentation that occurs in the active yeast, there can be fewer fructans in the bread. There are a number of people who can tolerate sourdough bread better than other bread.

28-Day Meal Plan

When looking at making a healthy change in eating habits, a meal plan can be the difference between success and failure. This section is aimed at helping kick-start the low-FODMAP diet. While the meal plan is used as an example, it is also intended to teach how this diet can be implemented. The plan is to put a structure in place to create a habit of healthy living. The menu can be changed easily by changing meals every 28 days. An example of this is switching a smoothie for breakfast on day 1 in the first 28-day cycle with a basil omelet on day 1 in the second cycle.
At the beginning of a diet, it can be extremely easy to cook food that is convenient, such as pre-cooked meals or to go to a restaurant or get fast food. These convenient meal sources can derail a diet before it has a chance to show any benefits.

Broadly speaking, a meal plan lays out what is for dinner a week or even 28 days before it is time to cook. There are three main components involved in meal planning: selecting meals and their recipes, shopping for ingredients, and preparing the ingredients. These components work in conjunction to benefit your health as well as your finances. Laying out a meal plan allows for healthy eating to be done on a budget; this creates a way to ensure that when life happens, the diet is not the first thing to get thrown out the door. However, before jumping into planning, it is important to understand the diet you are trying out and how to create a functional meal plan that suits your life.

The first thing to do is read up on the diet you are starting, which, in this context, will be the low-FODMAP diet. This knowledge creates the platform for removing high-FODMAP ingredients and reintroducing them in a controlled way.
After gaining a better knowledge of the diet, it is time to start constructing the first meal plan. To begin, it is a good idea to print out a sheet of paper that lays out the days of the week and has space to write down the meals that need to be planned; include meals that are not being eaten at home. With the week's plan laid out, the real work can begin.
It is time to decide on what will be eaten, including recipes. If you are planning for a family, it is fun to choose meals together to allow everyone to have a meal that they specifically want to eat. At first, the easiest thing to do may be to mainly plan dinners, marking down the difficulty of the recipes. Breakfasts and lunches can be partially planned until you have more confidence; however, this is only if you are easing into the diet. If you are eliminating all FODMAPS from the get-go, thoroughly planning out breakfasts and lunches is a good idea.

Once meals have been planned, the shopping list needs to be written. The easiest way to do this is to go through each meal and write down what ingredients are needed. These lists are best done once a week so that the ingredients you are using are fresh. Having fresh ingredients is ideal as this increases the nutrients you get with each meal. While there are many ingredients, like fruits and vegetables, that should be bought weekly, there are a few ingredients that can be stocked to cut costs. Some ingredients that can be stocked are sugar, flour, oils, and frozen produce.

Meal planning does not just help with eating healthy; the planning that is involved creates other benefits. Having a menu planned will lower the amount of stress in day-to-day life. You also save time because you already know what to buy and what needs to be cooked. To help save more time, it can be useful to prepare parts of the meals at the beginning of the week. This can be done by preparing and portioning out the meat and vegetables.

For many people, meals become boring because they end up eating the same dishes. When creating a meal plan, there is a small chance of dishes being overly repeated. By adding new dishes into your diet, there is an improvement in digestion as the different nutrients are introduced into the body. With each meal set out, it is also easier to prevent food waste. By planning out portions, the ingredients are used with minimum waste, which saves money spent on more ingredients.

A tip to save money and create less waste is to plan backward. At the end of a week or month, it is a good idea to look at what ingredients you still have in your fridge and freezer. Using these ingredients, you can create a menu that first uses the ingredients you still have before you do a shopping trip for the week.

The biggest tip for meal planning is to develop a routine. Developing a routine will make it easier to eat healthily and improve your overall lifestyle.

Meal Plan

This menu serves as a visual aid of what meals will be eaten when. It must be noted that recipes can be swapped with different meals to create a more balanced menu. This first menu lays out the meals in a simple but not strict manner. This allows for the development of the diet as time goes by. As menus, the two examples do not look at the strict serving information; they are guidelines to work from. The first menu gives not only the meals but also the way to plan a shopping list.

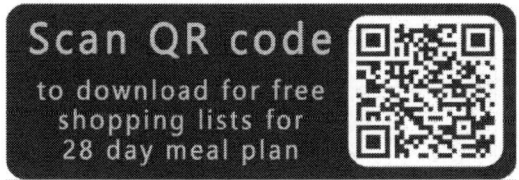

Week 1

Menu 1

DAY	1	2	3	4	5	6	7
Breakfast	Basic Smoothie Berry pag.142	Tomato omelet pag. 46	Quinoa porridge pag. 51	Green smoothie pag. 60	Egg wrap pag. 44	Peanut butter bowl pag. 50	Fluffy pancakes pag. 181
Lunch	Chicken wrap pag. 72	Corn Salad pag. 66	Rice paper spring rolls pag. 118	Hawaiian toasted Sandwich pag. 71	Carrot & walnut salad pag. 64	Thai noodle soup pag. 69	Tropical smoothie pag. 149
Dinner	Coconut crusted fish pag. 86	Baked chicken alfredo pag. 94	Bolognese pag. 88	Tofu Skewers pag. 92	Burgers pag. 96	Lamb stew pag. 98	Cheesy chicken pag. 84
Snack	Vegetable chips pag. 168		Salted caramel pumpkin seed pag. 165				Summer popsicles pag. 163
Drinks	8 cups Water	8 cups Water	8 cups Water	8 cups Water	8 cups Water	8 cups Water	8 cups Water

Menu 2

DAY	1	2	3	4	5	6	7
Breakfast	Breakfast warp pag. 48	Banana oatcakes pag. 52	Cranberry almond bowl pag. 155	Tomato omelet pag. 46	Crepes pag. 55	Baked oat cup pag. 169	Kale ginger pineapple smoothie pag. 145
Lunch	Smoothie basic strawberry pag.142	Quiche in ham cups pag.74	Pesto noodles pag.70	Corn on the cob pag.110	Carrot & walnut salad pag. 64	Chicken wrap pag. 72	Savory muffin pag. 75
Dinner	Bolognese pag. 88	Tune bacon quinoa bowl pag. 100	Tofu Skewers pag. 92	Cheesy chicken pag. 84	Minestrone pag. 89	Lamb stew pag. 98	Fried rice pag. 99
Snack		Sweet & savory popcorn pag. 158					
Drinks	8 cups Water	8 cups Water	8 cups Water	8 cups Water	8 cups Water	8 cups Water	8 cups Water

Shopping List for Week 1 (Menu 1)

Vegetables
- 2 bunches baby spinach
- 1 bunch kale
- 12 tomatoes
- 25 cherry tomatoes
- 6 cucumbers (3 small, 3 large)
- 1 red capsicum
- 2 heads of lettuce
- 22 carrots
- 1 parsnip
- 5 potatoes
- 1 red cabbage
- 5 spring onions
- ⅓ lb green beans
- 1 head of broccoli

Fruit
- 3 bananas
- 16 oz strawberries
- 1 pineapple
- 1 can of pineapple
- 5 limes
- 6 lemons
- 6 oranges
- 16 oz mixed berries
- ¼ cup dried, shredded coconut
- 4 oz olives

Protein
- 8 eggs
- 1 lb lamb, deboned
- 1 lb white fish
- 12 chicken breast fillets
- 2 lbs lean ground beef
- 6 ham slices

Dairy
- 1 pt Greek yogurt
- 2 pts almond milk
- 2 pts oat milk
- 2 cans coconut milk
- 1 bottle mayonnaise
- 1 block butter
- 1 block cheddar
- 1 block Parmesan
- 10 slices mozzarella

Grains
- ⅓ cup flaxseed
- 2 lbs gluten-free flour
- 1 packet gluten-free pasta
- ½ lb pumpkin seeds
- ½ lb walnuts
- ½ lb pecans
- ½ lb chestnuts
- ½ lb quinoa, uncooked
- 1 packet rice noodles
- 4 gluten-free wraps
- 1 loaf gluten-free bread
- ½ dozen gluten-free buns
- 12 rice paper wrappers

Condiments
- 1 jar smooth peanut butter
- 1 jar maple syrup
- 1 can miso paste
- 1 bottle soy sauce
- 2 cans tomato purée
- 1 can tomato paste

Sweeteners
- ¾ cup vanilla extract
- 1 lb white sugar
- 1 lb brown sugar

Herbs & spices
- 2 mild green chilis
- 1 bunch mint
- ¾ cup ginger, ground and crushed
- ¾ cup basil, fried
- 1 bunch fresh basil
- 8 lime leaves
- ¾ cup cinnamon, ground
- ¾ cup nutmeg, ground
- ¾ cup cumin
- 2 bunches cilantro
- 4 tbsp chili flakes
- 1 bunch sage
- ¾ cup oregano, dried

Liquids
- ½ cup vegetable stock, no garlic or onion

Oils
- 1 bottle olive oil
- 1 bottle sunflower oil
- 1 bottle garlic-infused oil
- 1 bottle Worcestershire sauce

Dry baking ingredients
- 1 ½ lbs powdered sugar

Week 2

Menu 1

DAY	8	9	10	11	12	13	14
Breakfast	Scrambled Tofu pag. 49	2 energy bars pag. 170	Smoothie bowl pag. 144	Crepes pag. 55	Basil omelet pag. 45	Kale ginger pineapple smoothie pag. 145	Quinoa muffin pag. 149
Lunch	Quiche in ham cups pag.74	Corn on the cob pag.110	Pesto sandwich pag.73	Tomato & green bean salad pag. 65	Smoothie basic coconut pag.142	Leftover Frittata pag. 90	Pineapple & yogurt rice cakes pag. 164
Dinner	Zucchini fritters pag. 112	Pork tacos pag. 85	Fresh vegetables & beetroot dip pag. 122	Fried rice pag. 99	Frittata pag. 90	Tuna, bacon quinoa bowl pag. 100	Pesto noodles pag.70
Snack			chia pudding pag. 174				strawberry ice cream pag. 186
Drinks	8 cups Water	8 cups Water	8 cups Water	8 cups Water	8 cups Water	8 cups Water	8 cups Water

Menu 2

DAY	8	9	10	11	12	13	14
Breakfast	Green smoothie pag. 60	Berry crumble pag. 175	Smoothie basic tropical pag.142	Energy bars pag. 170	Scrambled Tofu pag. 49	Electrolyte energizer pag. 128	Peanut butter bowl pag. 50
Lunch	Thai noodle soup pag. 69	Summer popsicles pag. 163	Chive dip & fresh vegetables (approved) pag. 120	Pesto noodles pag.70	Pineapple & yogurt rice cakes pag. 164	Quinoa muffin pag. 149	Corn Salad pag. 66
Dinner	Chicken fritters pag. 117	Frittata pag. 90	Lamb stew pag. 98	Cheesy chicken pag. 84	Fluffy pancakes & bacon pag. 181	Coconut crusted fish pag. 86	Baked chicken alfredo pag. 94
Snack			Coconut bites pag. 167				
Drinks	8 cups Water	8 cups Water	8 cups Water	8 cups Water	8 cups Water	8 cups Water	8 cups Water

Shopping List for Week 2 (Menu 1)

Vegetables
- 6 tomatoes
- 2 spring onions
- 1 head of lettuce
- 1 bunch kale
- 12 carrots
- 2 cucumbers (1 small, 1 large)
- 2 zucchinis
- ½ lb green beans
- 20 cherry tomatoes
- 2 red bell peppers
- ½ lb sweet potatoes
- ¼ lb leeks
- 6 ears of corn
- 1 head of broccoli

Fruit
- 14 bananas
- 7 oz strawberries
- 4 oz mixed berries
- 4 oz cranberries
- 3 limes
- 1 orange
- 1 can of pineapple
- 1 lemon

Protein
- 2 dozen eggs
- ½ lb pork loin
- 2 chicken breast fillets
- 6 ham slices
- ½ lb bacon
- 1 can shredded tuna in brine
- 5 oz firm tofu

Dairy
- 1 pt Greek yogurt
- ¾ pt coconut yogurt
- 1 can coconut milk
- ½ cup dark chocolate
- ½ cup mozzarella cheese
- 1 pt lactose-free milk

Grains
- ½ lb gluten-free oat flour
- 1 loaf gluten-free bread
- ½ lb rice flour
- 6 corn tortillas
- Rice cakes
- ¾ lb uncooked rice
- 1 packet rice noodles
- 1 cup quinoa flakes
- 1 lb puffed rice
- ¾ cup pumpkin seeds

Condiments
- 1 jar Dijon mustard
- ⅔ cup red wine vinegar
- 6 oz pesto, no garlic or onion

Sweeteners
None

Herbs & spices
- ¾ cup chives
- 1 cup chia seeds
- ¾ cup smoked paprika
- 1 jalapeño
- ¾ cup turmeric, ground

Liquids
None

Oils
- 1 bottle sesame oil
- 1 bottle rice vinegar

Dry baking ingredients
None

Week 3

Menu 1

DAY	15	16	17	18	19	20	21
Breakfast	Banana oatcakes **pag. 52**	Blueberry muffin **pag. 162**	Rhubarb granola bowl **pag. 54**	Fruit salad smoothie **pag. 153**	Basil omelet **pag. 45**	French toast casserole **pag. 53**	Hot ginger & lemon drink **pag. 132**
Lunch	Ham salad **pag. 67**	Chicken fritters **pag. 117**	Pumpkin cornbread & condiment of choice **pag. 113**	Lemon bar **pag. 189**	Garden medley **pag. 111**	Green smoothie **pag. 60**	Leftover Bolognese **pag. 88**
Dinner	Minestrone **pag. 89**	Fried rice **pag. 99**	Cheesy chicken **pag. 84**	Tofu Skewers **pag. 92**	Burgers **pag. 96**	Bolognese **pag. 88**	Hawaiian toasted Sandwich **pag. 71**
Snack				Energy bites **pag. 161**			
Drinks	8 cups Water	8 cups Water	8 cups Water	8 cups Water	8 cups Water	8 cups Water	8 cups Water

Menu 2

DAY	15	16	17	18	19	20	21
Breakfast	Rhubarb granola bowl **pag. 54**	Smoothie basic coconut **pag. 142**	Basil omelet **pag. 45**	Blueberry muffin **pag. 162**	Smoothie bowl **pag. 144**	Crepes **pag. 55**	Coconut bites **pag. 167**
Lunch	Vegetable chips **pag. 168**	Ham salad **pag. 67**	Tomato & green bean salad **pag. 65**	Garden medley **pag. 111**	Sweet & savory popcorn **pag. 158**	Hawaiian toasted Sandwich **pag. 71**	Beetroot dip cold cuts **pag. 122** & rice cake **pag. 164**
Dinner	Zucchini fritters **pag. 112**	Burgers **pag. 96**	Pork tacos **pag. 85**	Rice paper spring rolls **pag. 118**	Egg wrap **pag. 44**	Tofu Skewers **pag. 92**	Pesto noodles **pag. 70**
Snack					Baked oat cup **pag. 169**		
Drinks	8 cups Water	8 cups Water	8 cups Water	8 cups Water	8 cups Water	8 cups Water	8 cups Water

Shopping List for Week 3 (Menu 1)

Vegetables

- 10 tomatoes
- 20 carrots
- 2 cucumbers
- 1 yellow squash
- 1 green pepper
- 10 spring onions
- 4 cans crushed tomatoes
- 3 bunches baby spinach
- 1 bunch kale
- 1 bunch arugula
- 3 cans chickpeas in brine
- 1 pumpkin
- 1 potato
- ½ lb green beans
- 2 heads of lettuce
- 2 bell peppers
- 2 zucchinis

Fruit

- 2 bananas
- 1 lb cranberries
- 2 ½ lbs blueberries
- 1 lb rhubarb
- 1 lb mixed berries
- 4 lemons
- 1 pineapple
- 2 oranges
- 1 can fruit salad

Protein

- 12 eggs
- 4 chicken breast fillets
- 6 slices ham
- 2 lbs ground beef
- ½ lb firm tofu

Dairy

- ¾ cup mozzarella
- 1 ¼ cup feta
- 1 pt Greek yogurt
- ½ cup lactose-free yogurt
- 1 cup soy milk
- ½ cup dark chocolate
- 4 ½ sticks of butter, unsalted

Grains

- 1 loaf gluten-free bread
- ¾ cup pumpkin seeds
- ½ cup peanuts
- 1 packet gluten-free pasta shells
- 1 ¼ cups oats
- 1 packet gluten-free pasta
- Half dozen gluten-free buns
- 15 macadamia nuts
- 1 lb mixed nuts

Condiments

- 1 jar smooth peanut butter

Sweeteners

None

Herbs & spices

None

Liquids

None

Oils

None

Dry baking ingredients

None

Week 4

Menu 1

DAY	22	23	24	25	26	27	28
Breakfast	Banana porridge **pag. 47**	Pineapple strawberry raspberry smoothie **pag. 148**	Tomato omelet **pag. 46**	Baked oat cup **pag. 169**	Peanut butter bowl **pag. 50**	Chocolate protein smoothie **pag. 154**	Egg wrap **pag. 44**
Lunch	Carrot & walnut salad **pag. 64**	Thai noodle soup **pag. 69**	Quinoa muffin **pag. 149**	Pesto sandwich **pag.73**	Chicken wrap **pag. 72**	Vegetable chips **pag. 168**	Corn Salad **pag. 66**
Dinner	Pork tacos **pag. 85**	Lamb stew **pag. 98**	Coconut crusted fish **pag. 86**	Fried rice **pag. 99**	Pesto noodles **pag.70**	Baked chicken alfredo **pag. 94**	Frittata **pag. 90**
Snack		Summer popsicles **pag. 163**			Sweet & savory popcorn **pag. 158**		
Drinks	8 cups Water	8 cups Water	8 cups Water	8 cups Water	8 cups Water	8 cups Water	8 cups Water

Menu 2

DAY	22	23	24	25	26	27	28
Breakfast	Golden coffee **pag. 135**	PB&J cake in mug **pag. 188**	Egg wrap **pag. 44**	Chocolate energy bites **pag. 161**	Summer popsicles **pag. 163**	Quinoa porridge **pag. 51**	Chocolate protein smoothie **pag. 154**
Lunch	Chicken wrap **pag. 72**	Pineapple & yogurt rice cakes **pag. 164**	Salted caramel pumpkin seed **pag. 165**	Quiche in ham cups **pag.74**	Bread & vegetable dip **pag. 114**	Hot ginger & lemon drink **pag. 132**	Leftover Frittata **pag. 90**
Dinner	Bolognese **pag. 88**	Minestrone **pag. 89**	Tuna, bacon quinoa bowl **pag. 100**	Cheesy chicken **pag. 84**	Frittata **pag. 90**	Chicken fritters **pag. 117**	French toast casserole **pag. 53**
Snack	Vegetable chips **pag. 168**				Energy bar **pag. 170**		
Drinks	8 cups Water	8 cups Water	8 cups Water	8 cups Water	8 cups Water	8 cups Water	8 cups Water

Shopping List for Week 4 (Menu 1)

Vegetables
- 10 tomatoes
- 2 heads of lettuce
- 20 carrots
- 1 parsnip
- 2 sweet potatoes
- 8 potatoes
- 1 bunch baby spinach
- 14 oz cherry tomatoes
- 1 can corn
- 3 cucumbers
- 1 red capsicum
- 4 bell peppers
- 2 heads of broccoli
- 1 ¼ lbs green beans
- 12 spring onions
- 4 leeks
- 1 zucchini
- 1 pumpkin

Fruit
- 12 bananas
- 4 oz strawberries
- 2 oz pineapple
- 4 oz raspberries
- 4 oranges
- 1 lemon
- 2 limes
- 1 pineapple

Protein
- 12 eggs
- 1 lb lamb, deboned
- ½ pound white fish
- 1 lb pork loin
- 1 ½ lbs chicken

Dairy
- ⅔ pt almond milk
- 1 can coconut milk
- ½ cup cheddar cheese
- 1 pt Greek yogurt
- ¾ cup Parmesan cheese
- ½ cup mozzarella

Grains
- 2 packets rice noodles
- 4 gluten-free wraps
- 1 loaf gluten-free bread
- 1 ¼ cup popcorn kernels

Condiments
- 1 can pesto

Sweeteners
None

Herbs & spices
- 1 jalapeño
- 5 lime leaves

Liquids
- 1 ¼ cup protein powder
- ½ cup hot chocolate

Oils
None

Dry baking ingredients
None

Staple ingredients

Each week, it is a good idea to buy the fresh produce needed. There are some staple ingredients that are good to keep in stock.

Vegetables
- Tomatoes
- Cucumbers
- Lettuce
- Carrots
- Potatoes
- Spring onions

Fruit
- Bananas
- Mixed berries
- Oranges
- Lime
- Lemon

Protein
- Eggs
- Chicken breast fillets
- Lean ground beef

Dairy
- Lactose-free milk
- Almond milk
- Coconut milk
- Butter
- Mayonnaise
- Cheese, cheddar and Parmesan

Grains
- Gluten-free flour
- Mixed nuts
- Quinoa
- Rice noodles
- Approved pastas
- Gluten-free bread

Condiments
- Smooth peanut butter
- Maple syrup
- Soy sauce
- Tomato purée
- Worcestershire sauce

Sweeteners
- White sugar
- Brown sugar
- Vanilla extract

Herbs & spices
- Mint
- Ginger, ground and crushed
- Basil, fresh and dried
- Cinnamon, ground
- Cilantro, ground
- Sage, fresh and ground
- Oregano, fresh and ground
- Rosemary, fresh and ground

Liquids
- Soda water

Oils
- Olive oil
- Sunflower oil
- Garlic-infused oil

Dry baking ingredients
- Baking powder
- Baking soda
- Powdered sugar
- Cocoa powder

At the beginning of week one, go through the recipes in the meal plan. While going through the plan, begin writing a list, adding onto the staples list. Add in ingredients for snacks to eat during the week. For the next few weeks, create lists that build on each other. This is good practice for backward plan shopping trips in the future.

MEASUREMENT CONVERSIONS

Volume equivalents (Liquid)

US standard	US Ounces	Metric (approximate)
2 tablespoons	1 fl. Oz.	30 mL
¼ cup	2 fl. Oz.	60 mL
½ cup	4 fl. Oz.	120 mL
1 cup	8 fl. Oz.	240 mL
1½ cup	12 fl. Oz.	355 mL
2 cups or 1 pint	16 fl. Oz.	475 mL
4 cups or 1 quart	32 fl. Oz.	1 L
1 gallon	128 fl. Oz.	4 L

Volume equivalents (Dry)

US standard	Metric (approximate)
⅛ teaspoon	0.5 mL
¼ teaspoon	1 mL
½ teaspoon	2 mL
¾ teaspoon	4 mL
1 teaspoon	5 mL
1 tablespoon	15 mL
¼ cup	59 mL
⅓ cup	79 mL
½ cup	118 mL
⅔ cup	156 mL
¾ cup	177 mL
1 cup	235 mL
2 cups or 1 pint	475 mL
3 cups	700 mL
4 cups or 1 quart	1 L

Oven Temperatures	
Fahrenheit	Celsius (approximate)
250° F	120° C
300° F	150° C
325° F	165° C
350° F	180° C
375° F	190° C
400° F	200° C
425° F	220° C
450° F	230° C

Weight Equivalents	
US Standard	Metric (approximate)
½ ounce	15 g
1 ounce	30 g
2 ounces	60 g
4 ounces	115 g
8 ounces	225 g
12 ounces	340 g
16 ounces or 1 pound	455 g

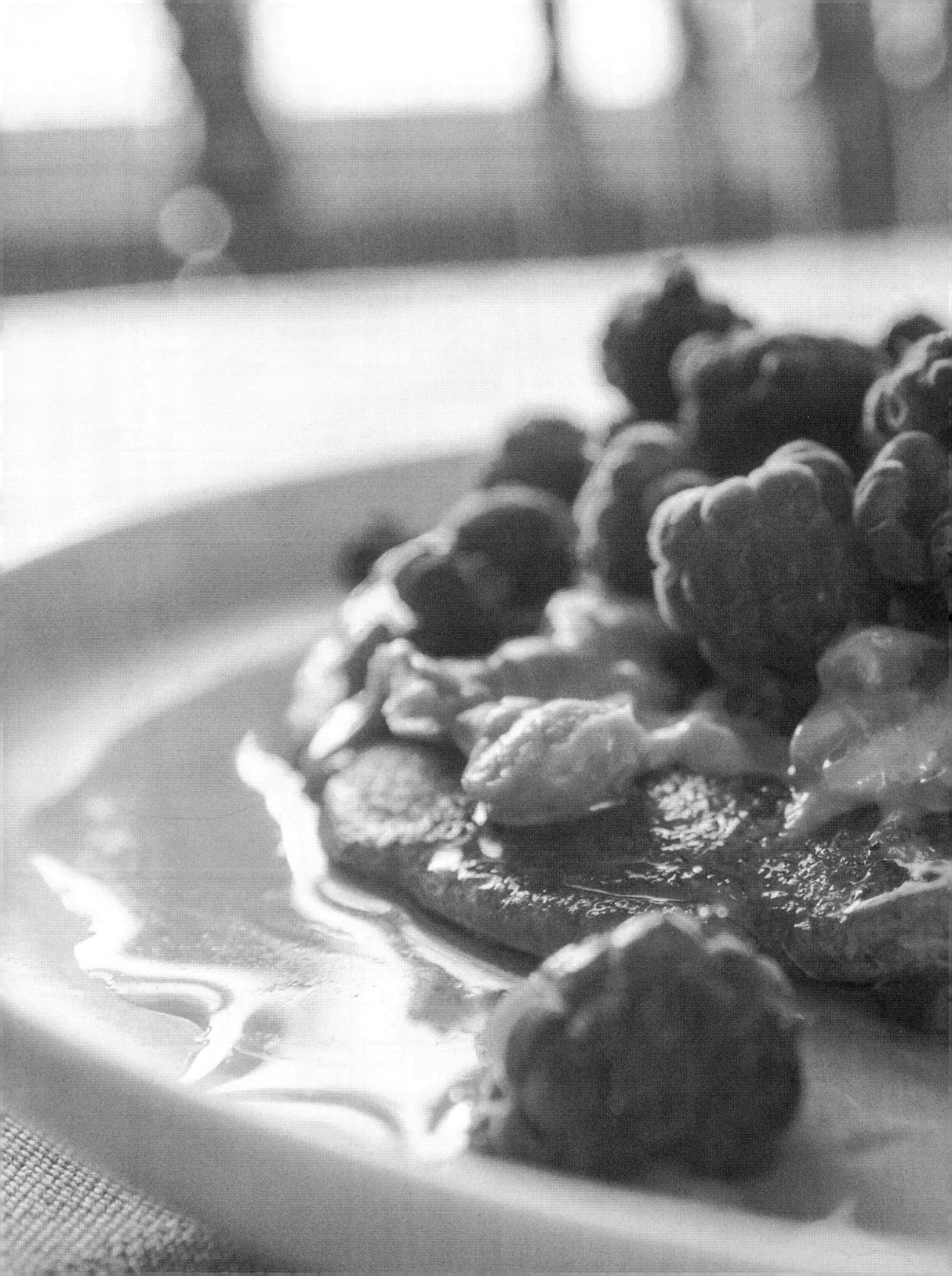

Breakfast

Egg Wraps **VEGETARIAN** 44

Basil Omelet with Smashed Tomato **VEGETARIAN** 45

Tomato Omelet **VEGETARIAN** 46

Banana Porridge **VEGAN** 47

Breakfast Wrap **VEGETARIAN** 48

Scrambled Tofu **VEGAN** 49

Peanut Butter Bowl **VEGETARIAN** 50

Quinoa Porridge **VEGAN** 51

Banana Oatcakes **VEGETARIAN** 52

French Toast Casserole **VEGAN** 53

Rhubarb Ginger Granola Bowl **VEGETARIAN** 54

Crepes and Berries **VEGETARIAN** 55

Carrot Cake Porridge **VEGAN** 56

Summer Berry Smoothie **VEGETARIAN** 57

Mixed Berry & Yogurt Granola Bar **VEGETARIAN** 58

Breakfast Tortillas **VEGETARIAN** 59

Green Smoothie **VEGETARIAN** 60

Egg Wraps

Cal 414
VEGETARIAN

Difficulty: Easy
Preparation time: 5 minutes
Cook time: 5 minutes
Servings: 4

Nutrition per serving (g)

Fat	Saturates	Carbs	Sugars	Fiber	Protein	Salt
33	8	2	2	0	25	0.2

Ingredients

- Oil to grease the pan (from the approved food list: avocado, olive, or sunflower)
- 4-8 eggs
- Pinch of salt
- Pepper

Method

1. Grease a non-stick pan with oil then place over medium heat to warm.

2. Whisk the egg in a bowl and pour it into the pan, ensuring it is spread evenly. Add in salt and pepper to taste.

3. Cook for 30-60 seconds on each side; gently flip when the edges on the first side are cooked.

4. Place on a plate to cool and repeat with the remainder of the eggs.

Tip

When using a small or medium pan (6-8 inches), cook one egg at a time. If using a large pan (10-12 inches), cook 2 eggs at a time.

Basil Omelet with Smashed Tomato

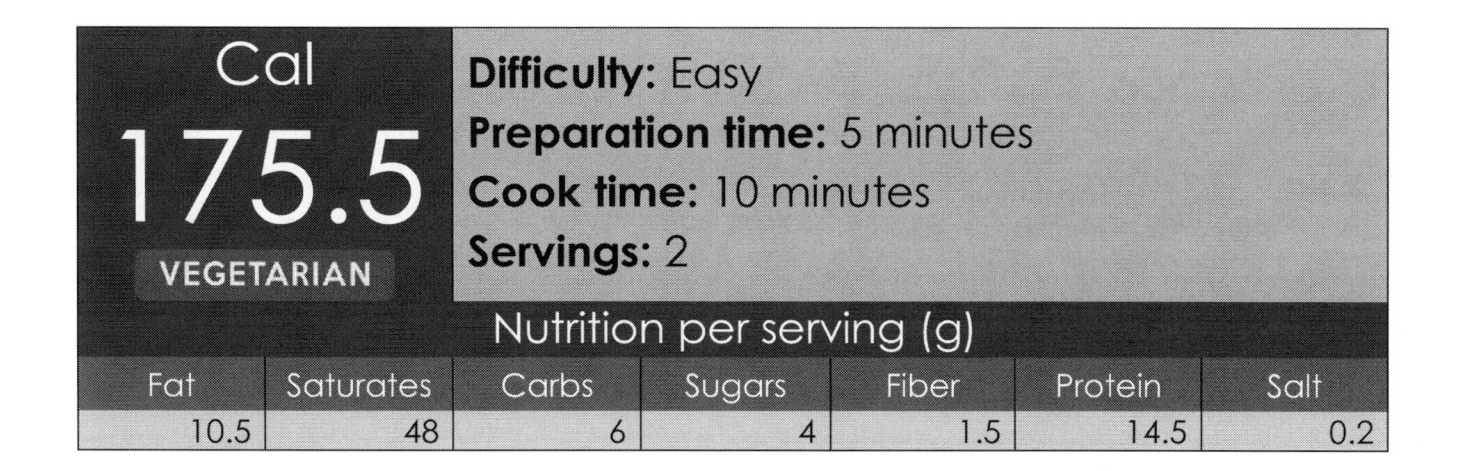

Cal 175.5 VEGETARIAN

Difficulty: Easy
Preparation time: 5 minutes
Cook time: 10 minutes
Servings: 2

Nutrition per serving (g)

Fat	Saturates	Carbs	Sugars	Fiber	Protein	Salt
10.5	48	6	4	1.5	14.5	0.2

Ingredients

- 2 tomatoes, halved
- 3 eggs
- 1 tbsp chives, chopped
- ¼ cup shredded mozzarella cheese (or other FODMAP-approved cheese)
- 1-2 basil leaves, chopped finely
- Pepper

Method

1 Break the eggs into a bowl and add a splash of water. Whisk the mixture with a fork and add the chives and a pinch of pepper. Set aside.

2 Place the halved tomatoes on tinfoil in a hot skillet on the stove or onto a hot grill on low to medium heat. Turn occasionally until they are starting to char, then remove them and place them on plates. Squish slightly so that the juices are released.

3 Take the egg mixture and whisk it slightly before pouring it into a hot pan on medium heat. Leave the mixture for a few seconds before gently stirring the uncooked egg until it is cooked but still slightly loose.

4 Place the cheese and a basil leaf on one half of the egg and then gently fold the omelet in half. Let it cook for another minute. Once it is cooked, cut the omelet in half and serve with the tomato.

Tomato Omelet

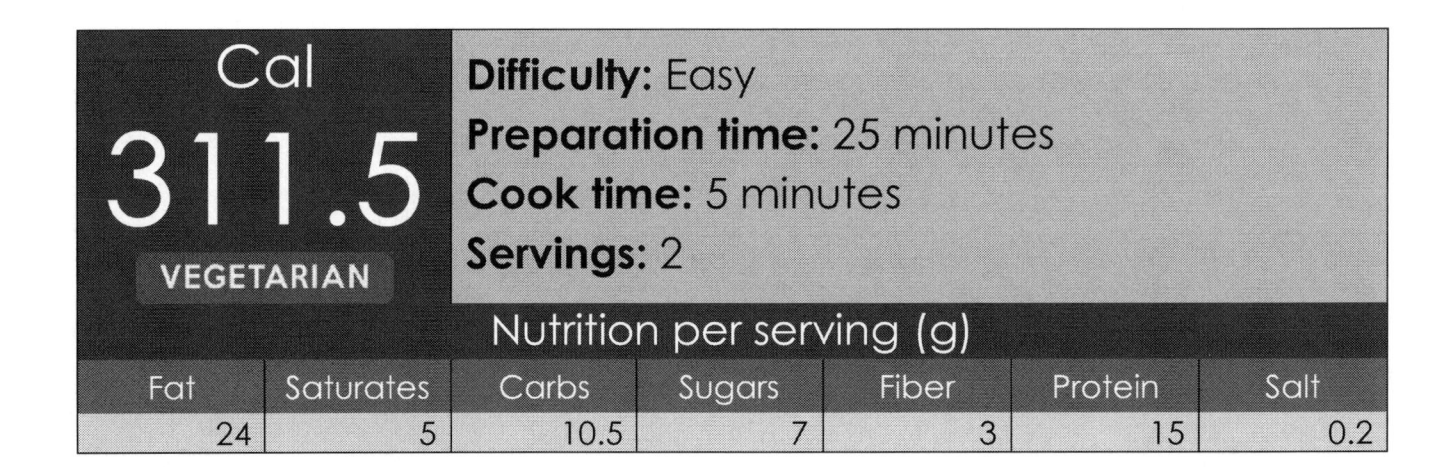

Cal 311.5 — VEGETARIAN

Difficulty: Easy
Preparation time: 25 minutes
Cook time: 5 minutes
Servings: 2

Nutrition per serving (g)

Fat	Saturates	Carbs	Sugars	Fiber	Protein	Salt
24	5	10.5	7	3	15	0.2

Ingredients

- 4 fresh tomatoes
- 4 eggs
- ¼ cup water
- ½ tsp chopped basil
- Pinch of salt
- Pinch of pepper
- 2 tbsp olive oil (or other approved oil)

Method

1. Place a pot of water on the stove and bring to a boil. Mark each tomato with an 'x' in the skin and place them in the water. Leave the tomatoes in the water for 30 seconds before removing them with a draining spoon and placing them into cold water.

2. Peel the skin off the tomatoes and cut them in half. Remove the core and seeds and slice into strips. Set them aside.

3. Break the eggs into a bowl and whisk together while adding the basil, salt, and pepper. Stop whisking when the mixture is frothy. Place the mixture into a hot pan that has been greased with oil.

4. Gently stir the mixture while cooking over medium heat. When the mixture starts to get firm, spread the tomato over it. Do not continue stirring the mixture. When the tomatoes are warmed through, remove from the pan and enjoy.

Banana Porridge

Cal 450
VEGAN

Difficulty: Easy
Preparation time: 2 minutes
Cook time: 5 minutes
Servings: 1

Nutrition per serving (g)

Fat	Saturates	Carbs	Sugars	Fiber	Protein	Salt
14.7	1.4	73.3	25.4	7.6	7.8	0.2

Ingredients

- ½ cup rolled oats
- ½ cup almond milk
- ⅓ cup banana, sliced
- 2 tsp sunflower oil
- 2 tsp maple syrup
- ¼ tsp vanilla extract
- Pinch of cinnamon

Method

1. Cook the oats according to the instructions and use almond milk.

2. Combine oil, syrup, cinnamon, and vanilla in a saucepan over medium heat. Let the mixture bubble for a minute and add the banana. Cook for 3 minutes. The banana should look plump.

3. Serve the oats with the banana on top.

Breakfast Wrap

Cal 247
VEGETARIAN

Difficulty: Easy
Preparation time: 4 minutes
Cook time: 3 minutes
Servings: 1

Nutrition per serving (g)

Fat	Saturates	Carbs	Sugars	Fiber	Protein	Salt
17	5	9.5	1.5	2.5	13.5	0.2

Ingredients

- Oil for frying pan (FODMAP-approved)
- 2 eggs
- 1 tsp garlic-infused oil (optional)
- 1 ½ tbsp chives, chopped
- 1 low-FODMAP gluten-free wrap
- ¼ cup of spinach
- ½ sliced tomato
- 2 tbsp FODMAP-approved cheese (shredded)

Method

1. Grease a frying pan with oil and place on medium heat.

2. In a bowl, mix the eggs, garlic-infused oil, and chives before pouring into the pan. Once the mixture starts to set, carefully flip it to cook the other side.

3. Heat the wrap according to the instructions on the packaging, and then place it onto a plate. Put the egg mixture on the wrap with enough of the wrap open so it can be rolled. Add the spinach, tomato, and cheese on top of the egg and roll the wrap.

Scrambled Tofu

Cal 82 VEGAN	**Difficulty:** Easy **Preparation time:** 5 minutes **Cook time:** 5 minutes **Servings:** 1

Nutrition per serving (g)

Fat	Saturates	Carbs	Sugars	Fiber	Protein	Salt
5	0.5	4	2	0.5	5	0.2

Ingredients

- ½ cup medium-firm tofu
- ¼ cup water
- 1 tbsp soy sauce
- ¼ tsp turmeric, ground
- ½ cup grated carrot and zucchini
- Oil for greasing the pan
- 1 slice FODMAP-approved bread

Method

1. In a bowl, thoroughly mix together the water, soy sauce, and turmeric. Once mixed, add the vegetables and crumble the tofu into the bowl.

2. Place an oil-greased pan onto medium heat and place the mixture in it. Fry the mixture for 5 minutes or until it is golden brown.

3. Serve with a slice of FODMAP-approved toast.

Peanut Butter Bowl

Cal 519
VEGETARIAN

Difficulty: Easy
Preparation time: 3 minutes
Cook time: 5 minutes
Servings: 2

Nutrition per serving (g)

Fat	Saturates	Carbs	Sugars	Fiber	Protein	Salt
35	13.5	5.5	25	5.5	15.5	0.2

Ingredients

- 2 bananas, chopped and frozen
- 1 ½ cups Greek yogurt
- 2 tbsp peanut butter
- ¼ cup chopped nuts

Method

1 In a blender, mix the bananas, yogurt, and peanut butter.

2 When the mixture is a smooth consistency, pour it into a bowl and top with chopped nuts.

3 Simple!

Quinoa Porridge

Cal 292 VEGAN

Difficulty: Easy
Preparation time: 2 minutes
Cook time: 25 minutes
Servings: 2

Nutrition per serving (g)

Fat	Saturates	Carbs	Sugars	Fiber	Protein	Salt
8	1.5	50.5	17	4.5	7.5	0.2

Ingredients

- ½ cup quinoa
- 1 tsp oil (FODMAP-approved)
- 1 cup water
- ¾ cup milk (FODMAP-approved)
- ¼ tsp cinnamon
- 2 tbsp maple syrup
- 1 cup berries (FODMAP-approved)

Method

1. Rinse the quinoa under cold water for two minutes using a fine sieve and then transfer it to a medium saucepan with oil. Toast the quinoa until the water has evaporated.

2. Add water to the saucepan and bring to a boil. Once the water starts boiling, turn the heat down to the lowest setting and cover with a lid. Cook for 12-15 minutes until the quinoa is fluffy. Drain the excess water and place the quinoa back into the saucepan.

3. Mix the cinnamon, milk, and syrup into the quinoa. If the milk evaporates, add a small amount as needed. Let the mix simmer for 5 minutes or until the mixture is warmed through.

4. Serve the mixture in a bowl with berries on top.

Banana Oatcakes

Cal 530
VEGETARIAN

Difficulty: Easy
Preparation time: 34 minutes
Cook time: 32 minutes
Servings: 4

Nutrition per serving (g)

Fat	Saturates	Carbs	Sugars	Fiber	Protein	Salt
12.5	2.75	80	5.5	14.5	21.25	0.2

Ingredients

- 1 unripe banana
- 1 egg
- ½ cup rice milk
- 1 tbsp Greek yogurt
- 1 ½ cups rolled oats
- ⅓ cup oat flour
- 2 tsp cinnamon
- Pinch of salt

Method

1. Mash the banana in a bowl and add the egg, milk, and yogurt, whisking after each ingredient. Next, add the dry ingredients, making sure to mix thoroughly.

2. Let the mixture rest for 15-30 minutes.

3. Grease a pan with low-FODMAP-approved oil and place it on medium heat.

4. Pour ¼ of the batter into the pan and flip when it begins bubbling. Remove the oatcake when it is golden brown on both sides.

5. Repeat 3 more times until you have 4 oatcakes.

6. Add a low-FODMAP-approved topping if desired.

French Toast Casserole

Cal 208 VEGAN

Difficulty: Medium
Preparation time: 15 minutes
Cook time: 1 hour
Servings: 8

Nutrition per serving (g)

Fat	Saturates	Carbs	Sugars	Fiber	Protein	Salt
2.75	0.8	41.6	9.75	2.25	3	0.2

Ingredients

- 1 banana
- ¼ cup maple syrup
- ½ cup chickpea water (drained from canned chickpeas in water)
- ¾ cup almond milk
- 1 tsp vanilla extract
- 1 tsp cinnamon
- 8 servings gluten-free bread, cut into 1-inch squares
- 2 cups mixed berries

Method

1. Mash the banana in a bowl and stir in the maple syrup.

2. In a separate bowl, whip the chickpea water into soft peaks with a hand mixer.

3. Mix the banana, vanilla extract, and cinnamon into the whipped chickpea water.

4. Grease a casserole dish and add the bread chunks. Pour the banana mixture over it while gently tossing it to cover all the bread.

5. Scatter the berries over the top and place in the fridge overnight

6. In the morning, place the mixture into an oven preheated to 350°F and bake for 50-60 minutes.

Rhubarb Ginger Granola Bowl

Cal 593
VEGETARIAN

Difficulty: Medium
Preparation time: 10 minutes
Cook time: 30 minutes
Servings: 4

Nutrition per serving (g)

Fat	Saturates	Carbs	Sugars	Fiber	Protein	Salt
4	1.5	32	19	4	20	0.2

Ingredients

Yogurt

- 1 ½ cups chopped rhubarb
- 1 tbsp grated ginger
- ½ tbsp lemon juice
- 4 tbsp maple syrup
- Pinch of salt
- 2 cups Greek yogurt

Granola

- ½ cup pumpkin seeds
- ¾ cup chopped nuts (low-FODMAP-approved)
- 2 tbsp melted coconut oil
- 1 tsp ground ginger
- ¼ tsp cinnamon
- Pinch of salt

Method

1. Preheat the oven to 350°F.

2. For the yogurt, in a small pot over medium heat, add chopped rhubarb, ginger, lemon juice, and 2 tablespoons of maple syrup. Stir the mixture occasionally until it begins to simmer, ensuring the bottom of the pot does not burn. Once the mixture has thickened to a purée consistency, mix in the other 2 tablespoons of maple syrup. Place the mixture into a bowl to cool.

3. Place the granola ingredients into a separate bowl and mix until the coconut oil coats everything. Move the mix onto a non-stick baking tray and place in the oven for 10-15 minutes, stirring halfway.

4. Once all components are ready, fold the rhubarb purée into the yogurt and sprinkle the granola over top. The yogurt can be stored in the fridge and the granola in a Tupperware.

5. Add a low-FODMAP-approved topping if desired.

Crepes and Berries

Cal 277 — VEGETARIAN

Difficulty: Easy
Preparation time: 18 minutes
Cook time: 8 minutes
Servings: 4

Nutrition per serving (g)

Fat	Saturates	Carbs	Sugars	Fiber	Protein	Salt
10.5	4.5	25	6	3.5	8	0.2

Ingredients

Crepes
- ½ cup oat flour
- 1 tsp brown sugar
- 1 tsp white sugar
- 2 eggs
- 1 ½ tbsp melted butter
- 1 tsp vanilla extract

Filling
- ½ cup berry mix
- Pinch of brown sugar
- Pinch of cinnamon
- 2 tbsp Greek yogurt

Method

1. In a blender, place the crepe ingredients and blend for two minutes. Set aside to rest for 15 minutes.

2. Mix the brown sugar and cinnamon with the berries.

3. After the crepe mix has rested, place a non-stick pan, greased with oil, over medium heat. Add ¼ cup of the crepe batter to the pan. Gently move the pan to cover the bottom of the pan with a thin layer of batter. Cook for a minute and gently flip.

4. Once the crepes are cooked, place them on a plate and top with a small amount of yogurt, fold, and place the berries on top.

Carrot Cake Porridge

Cal 290
VEGAN

Difficulty: Easy
Preparation time: 5 minutes
Cook time: 20 minutes
Servings: 4

Nutrition per serving (g)

Fat	Saturates	Carbs	Sugars	Fiber	Protein	Salt
9.6	2	29.5	12.3	5.6	9.6	0.3

Ingredients

- 1 cup oats
- 3 cups water
- 2 medium carrots, grated
- 1 tsp cinnamon
- 1 ½ tbsp flax seeds
- ¼ cup cranberries, dried
- ¼ cup walnuts
- ½ cup almond milk
- 1 tsp maple syrup

Method

1. Add the oats and water to a pot over medium heat. As it comes to a boil, turn the heat down and stir the carrots and cinnamon into the pot.

2. Cook for 10-12 minutes, until you reach the desired texture. Add the cranberries and nuts before serving.

Summer Berry Smoothie

Cal 406 VEGETARIAN	**Difficulty:** Easy **Preparation time:** 5 minutes **Cook time:** - **Servings:** 4					

Nutrition per serving (g)

Fat	Saturates	Carbs	Sugars	Fiber	Protein	Salt
3.3	1.6	10.7	10.7	0.8	5.8	0.3

Ingredients

- 1 large banana, unripe
- ¼ cup blueberries
- 1 ¼ cups lactose-free milk even vegetable milk (NO oat milk for gluten-free)
- 1 cup Greek yogurt
- Ice

Method

1. Place ingredients in a blender and mix until smooth.

Mixed Berry & Yogurt Granola Bar

Cal 784
VEGETARIAN

Difficulty: Easy
Preparation time: 5 minutes
Cook time: 30 minutes
Servings: 12

Nutrition per serving (g)

Fat	Saturates	Carbs	Sugars	Fiber	Protein	Salt
9.5	3.2	18.5	6.4	2.8	3.9	0.3

Ingredients

- 2 cups rolled oats
- 3 tbsp shredded coconut
- 2 tbsp macadamia nut meal
- 4 tbsp chia seeds
- 1 egg (whites only)
- ⅓ cup peanut oil
- ¼ cup maple syrup
- 1 cup mixed berries
- 1 ½ cups Greek yogurt
- 3 tbsp white chocolate, melted

Method

1. Preheat the oven to 375°F. Line a baking tray with parchment paper.

2. Mix the ingredients in a bowl, and then press into the pan. Bake for 30 minutes.

3. Allow to cool, then drizzle with chocolate and serve.

Breakfast Tortillas

Cal **373**
VEGETARIAN

Difficulty: Easy
Preparation time: 5 minutes
Cook time: 10 minutes
Servings: 4

Nutrition per serving (g)

Fat	Saturates	Carbs	Sugars	Fiber	Protein	Salt
19.5	9.75	19.75	6	3.75	19.5	0.2

Ingredients

- 4 corn tortillas
- 4 eggs
- ¼ cup macadamia nuts
- 1 cup mozzarella cheese, grated
- 1 cup Greek yogurt
- 4 tomatoes, diced

Method

1. Boil the uncracked eggs in simmering water for 5 ½ minutes, then place in cold water to stop cooking. Peel when they have cooled.

2. Heat tortillas on both sides for 20 seconds in a pan over medium heat. Place in an airtight container and cover with a dry cloth while heating the rest of the tortillas.

3. Spread the yogurt over the tortillas and add the cheese and tomatoes. Cut the eggs in half before adding them to the tortilla. Season to taste.

Green Smoothie

Cal **347** VEGETARIAN	**Difficulty:** Easy **Preparation time:** 5 minutes **Cook time:** 0 minutes **Servings:** 1

Nutrition per serving (g)

Fat	Saturates	Carbs	Sugars	Fiber	Protein	Salt
24	16	31	17	10	8	0.2

Ingredients

- ½ cup fresh pineapple, chopped and then frozen
- 2 tablespoons baby spinach
- ¼ cup Greek yogurt
- 1 tbsp shredded coconut
- 2 tsp chia seeds
- ¼ cup almond milk
- 6 ice cubes

Method

1. Blend all the ingredients, except for the ice and milk.
2. Add the ice and blend.
3. Add the milk and continue blending until smooth.

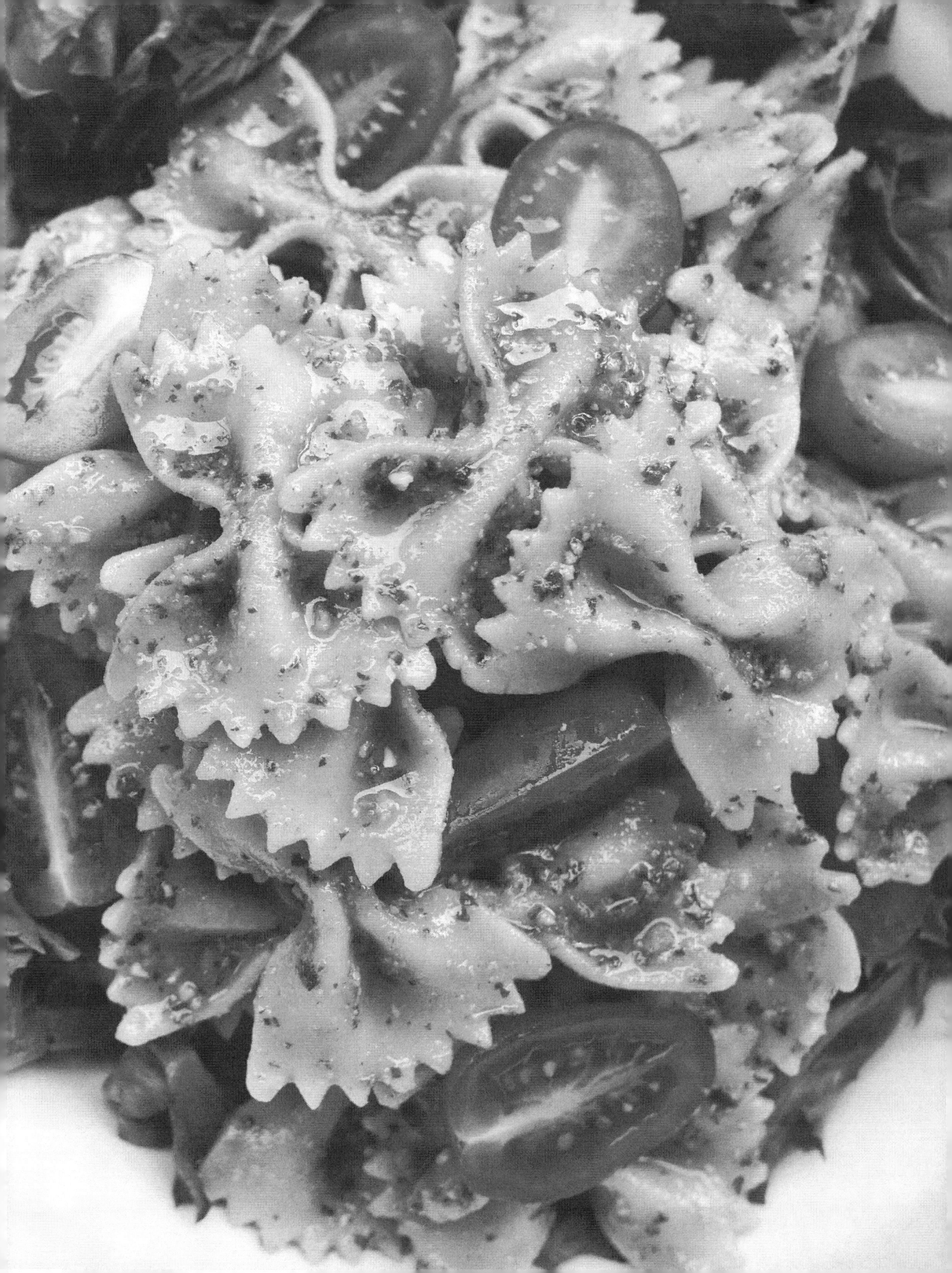

Lunch

Carrot and Walnut Salad `VEGAN` 64

Tomato and Green Bean Salad `VEGETARIAN` 65

Corn Salad `VEGAN` 66

Ham Salad 67

Basil Vinaigrette Salad Dressing `VEGAN` 68

Thai Pumpkin Noodle Soup `VEGAN` 69

Pesto Noodles `VEGETARIAN` 70

Hawaiian Toasted Sandwich 71

Chicken Wrap 72

Pesto Toasted Sandwich 73

Quiche in Ham Cups 74

Savory Muffins `VEGETARIAN` 75

Feta, Chicken, and Pepper Sandwich 76

Rice & Zucchini Slice `VEGETARIAN` 77

Cranberry Chocolate Chip Energy Bites `VEGAN` 78

Cucumber salad `VEGETARIAN` 79

Cheese, Ham, and Spinach Muffins 80

Carrot and Walnut Salad

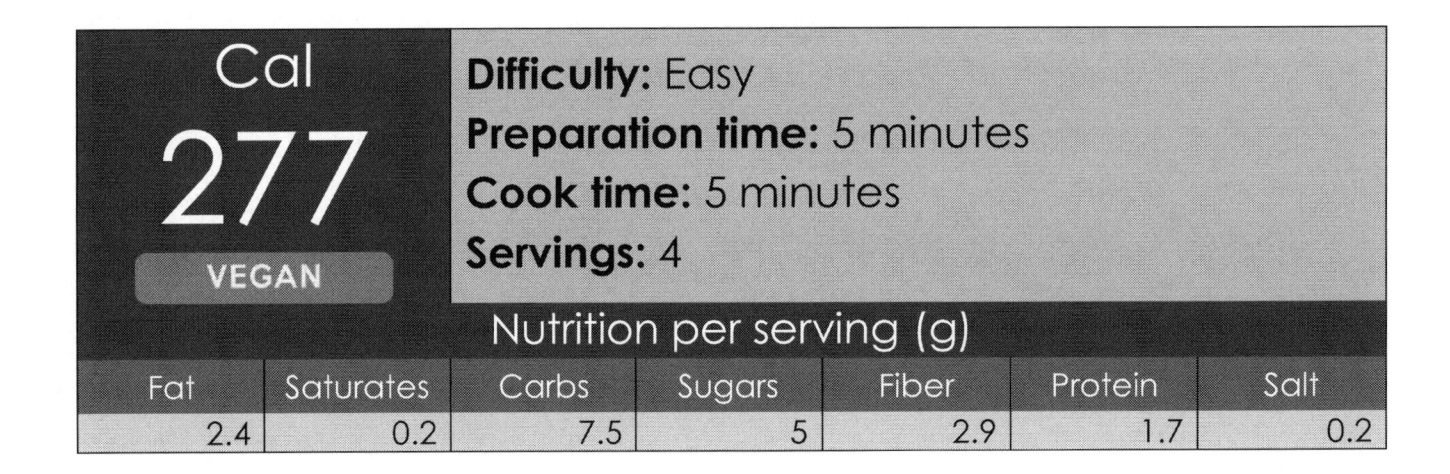

Cal 277
VEGAN

Difficulty: Easy
Preparation time: 5 minutes
Cook time: 5 minutes
Servings: 4

Nutrition per serving (g)

Fat	Saturates	Carbs	Sugars	Fiber	Protein	Salt
2.4	0.2	7.5	5	2.9	1.7	0.2

Ingredients

- ½ cup lettuce
- 3 carrots, peeled
- ¼ cup walnuts, chopped
- ¼ cup orange juice
- Pinch of salt

Method

1 Wash the lettuce and carrots, and then shred the lettuce into a bowl. Shave the carrots into strips and mix with the lettuce.

2 Place a greased pan over medium heat. Add the walnuts and fry quickly (2 minutes), stirring often to prevent the walnuts from burning. Remove the walnuts from the pan and place onto a paper towel. Sprinkle with salt.

3 Mix the lettuce and carrots in a bowl. Add the orange juice and the walnuts before serving.

Tomato and Green Bean Salad

Cal 125 — VEGETARIAN

Difficulty: Easy
Preparation time: 3 minutes
Cook time: 5 minutes
Servings: 6

Nutrition per serving (g)

Fat	Saturates	Carbs	Sugars	Fiber	Protein	Salt
8.8	2	10.8	4.5	1.8	2.5	0.5

Ingredients

- 1 cup green beans
- ½ cup mayonnaise
- ½ cup Greek yogurt
- 1 tbsp chopped basil
- 2 tbsp chopped parsley
- Pinch of salt
- Pinch of pepper
- 2 tbsp lactose-free or another FODMAP-approved milk
- 1 tbsp Dijon mustard
- 2 tomatoes
- 2 spring onions, green part only
- 1 ½ cups lettuce

Method

1 In a bowl, mix mayonnaise, yogurt, milk, mustard, basil, parsley, salt, and pepper.

2 Wash the green beans, lettuce, and spring onions, then drain the water and chop the green onions. Shred the lettuce into a separate bowl and mix in the green beans and spring onions.

3 Cut the tomatoes into quarters and mix into the bowl. Put the dressing into a serving jug and serve.

Corn Salad

Cal 189 VEGAN

Difficulty: Easy
Preparation time: 2 minutes
Cook time: 5 minutes
Servings: 2

Nutrition per serving (g)

Fat	Saturates	Carbs	Sugars	Fiber	Protein	Salt
8	1.5	17	10.5	5	5	0.5

Ingredients

- 1 can (15 oz) corn
- 1 cup cherry tomatoes
- 1 cup cucumber
- 2 spring onions, green parts only
- 1 red capsicum
- 2 tbsp mayonnaise (vegan)

Method

1. Slice the tomatoes in half.
2. Cut the cucumber into slices and then quarters. Chop the green part of the spring onion finely.
3. Thinly slice the capsicum.
4. Mix all the ingredients with the mayonnaise in a bowl and serve.

Ham Salad

Cal 576

Difficulty: Easy
Preparation time: 5 minutes
Cook time: 5 minutes
Servings: 2

Nutrition per serving (g)

Fat	Saturates	Carbs	Sugars	Fiber	Protein	Salt
48	24	5.5	2.5	2	31.5	0.3

Ingredients

Salad
- 2 cups baby spinach and arugula
- 25 blueberries
- 6 slices ham, cold cut, cut into small pieces
- 15 macadamia nuts, halved
- 1 cup feta cheese
- Pinch of salt
- Pinch of pepper

Dressing
- 1 tbsp rice vinegar
- 1 tbsp olive oil
- 1 tbsp maple syrup

Method

1. Place the salad ingredients, except for the feta and black pepper, into a bowl and set aside.

2. Mix the dressing ingredients in a small bowl, then pour over the salad. Cover the salad and shake until the dressing covers everything evenly. Crumble the feta into the bowl and add the pepper.

Basil Vinaigrette Salad Dressing

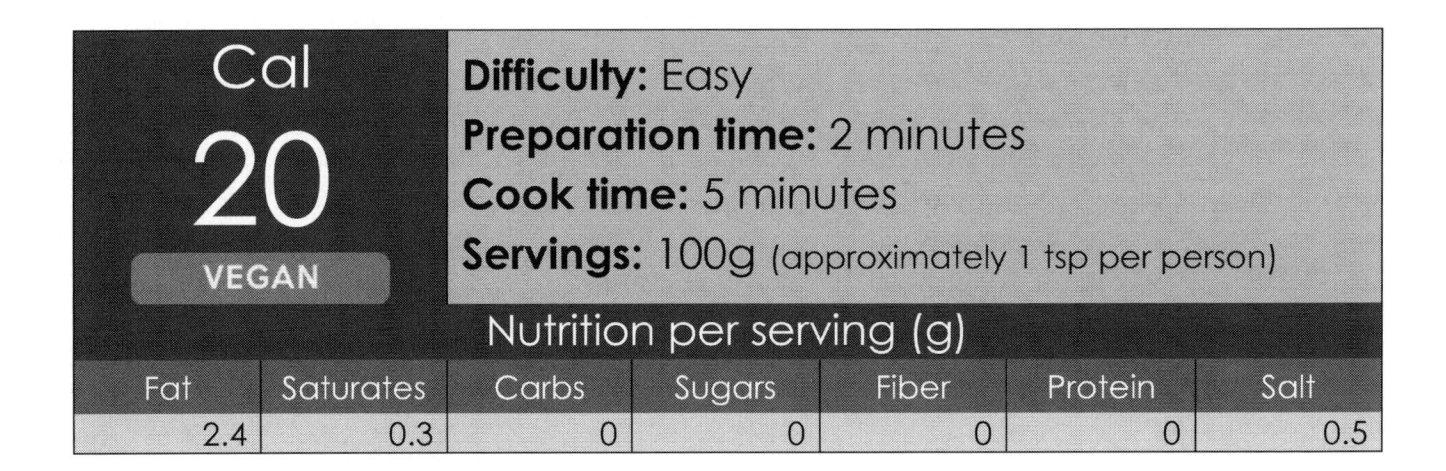

Cal 20
VEGAN

Difficulty: Easy
Preparation time: 2 minutes
Cook time: 5 minutes
Servings: 100g (approximately 1 tsp per person)

Nutrition per serving (g)

Fat	Saturates	Carbs	Sugars	Fiber	Protein	Salt
2.4	0.3	0	0	0	0	0.5

Ingredients

- 1 cup olive oil
- ½ cup white vinegar
- 1 tbsp basil, shredded
- 1 tbsp garlic-infused oil
- Pinch of salt
- Pinch of pepper

Method

1. In a bottle with a lid, add all the ingredients.
2. Shake the bottle to mix and then refrigerate.

Thai Pumpkin Noodle Soup

Cal 373 VEGAN

Difficulty: Easy
Preparation time: 10 minutes
Cook time: 55 minutes
Servings: 6

Nutrition per serving (g)

Fat	Saturates	Carbs	Sugars	Fiber	Protein	Salt
16.3	12.3	52.6	8.1	7.7	7.4	0.6

Ingredients

Roast vegetables

- 3 ¼ cups pumpkin, peeled, deseeded, and cubed
- 1 cup carrots, peeled and cubed
- 1 tsp cumin, ground
- 2 tsp olive oil
- Pinch of salt
- Pinch of pepper

Soup

- 2 cups vegetable stock, without garlic or onion
- 1 cup spring onions, green part only, chopped finely
- 1 tsp ginger, crushed
- ½ tsp lemon zest
- 2 tsp soy sauce
- Pinch of chili flakes, to taste
- 1 ½ cups coconut milk, canned
- 1 cup thin rice noodles
- ¼ cup cilantro

Method

1. Preheat the oven to 350°F. Place the peeled and cubed pumpkin and carrots onto a roasting tray. Use the oil to coat the vegetables and season with cumin, salt, and pepper. Bake for 20-30 minutes, turning halfway. Remove when the vegetables are soft and golden.

2. Set the vegetables aside to cool for 10 minutes, and then blend them together with the stock until smooth.

3. Over medium heat, heat a saucepan, add some oil, and fry the spring onion for 3 minutes. Add the ginger. Let cook for another minute before adding the pumpkin and coconut milk.

4. Stir in the lemon zest, soy sauce, and chili flakes. Allow the soup to simmer for 10 minutes on low heat. Add water if the soup seems too thick.

5. Cook the noodles according to the instructions on the packet while the soup cooks. When cooked, stir the noodles into the soup with cilantro and serve.

Pesto Noodles

Cal 569 VEGETARIAN

Difficulty: Easy
Preparation time: 5 minutes
Cook time: 10 minutes
Servings: 2

Nutrition per serving (g)

Fat	Saturates	Carbs	Sugars	Fiber	Protein	Salt
50	5.5	26	1.5	3	6	0.2

Ingredients

Pesto
- ¾ cup basil, fresh
- 2 tbsp garlic-infused oil
- ¼ cup pine nuts
- 2 tbsp olive oil
- Pinch of salt
- Pinch of pepper
- ½ cup Parmesan, grated

Noodles
- 1 cup rice noodles

Method

1. In a food processor, mix basil, garlic oil, and pine nuts until coarsely chopped.

2. Add the olive oil, cheese, salt, and pepper to the processor and mix until the pesto is fully mixed and smooth.

3. Cook the noodles according to the instructions on the packet. Once cooked, toss the noodles in a bowl with 3 tablespoons pesto and mix until the noodles are covered.

4. Serve!

Hawaiian Toasted Sandwich

Cal 454

Difficulty: Easy
Preparation time: 4 minutes
Cook time: 6 minutes
Servings: 1

Nutrition per serving (g)

Fat	Saturates	Carbs	Sugars	Fiber	Protein	Salt
26.5	9.9	33.7	3	1.8	19.9	1

Ingredients

- 2 slices bread
- 1 tbsp butter
- 2 ½ tbsp pineapple chunks, drained
- 2 slices cheddar cheese
- 2 slices ham, cold cut
- 1 tbsp spring onion, tips finely chopped
- Pinch of black pepper

Method

1. Place a frying pan over medium heat.
2. Spread butter on the outside of each slice of bread.
3. Prepare the filling by grating the cheese, slicing the ham, rinsing the pineapple, and chopping the spring onion finely.
4. Put the sandwich together adding pepper to taste and ensuring the butter is on the outside.
5. Place in the frying pan and cook each side for 3 minutes. The bread should turn golden brown.
6. Serve warm.

Chicken Wrap

Cal 392	**Difficulty:** Easy **Preparation time:** 5 minutes **Cook time:** 0 minutes **Servings:** 4

Nutrition per serving (g)

Fat	Saturates	Carbs	Sugars	Fiber	Protein	Salt
12.7	4.7	17.7	3.5	5.5	22.7	0.2

Ingredients

- 1 ½ cups chicken, cooked and chopped
- 3 cups lettuce, chopped
- 20 cherry tomatoes, halved
- ¼ cup Parmesan, grated
- Pinch of pepper
- 4 gluten-free wraps, can substitute with other low-FODMAP-approved wraps

Method

1. In a bowl, mix together all the ingredients, leaving the wraps to the side.

2. Lay the wraps out and place ¼ of the mixture onto the center. Roll up. If taking to eat on the go, use a toothpick to secure the wrap.

Pesto Toasted Sandwich

Cal 555

Difficulty: Easy
Preparation time: 5 minutes
Cook time: 5 minutes
Servings: 1

Nutrition per serving (g)

Fat	Saturates	Carbs	Sugars	Fiber	Protein	Salt
35	15	28	3	3	33	0.2

Ingredients

- 2 slices gluten-free bread
- 1 tbsp butter
- 1 tbsp pesto, no garlic or onion in the mixture
- 4 cherry tomatoes, halved
- 1 slice mozzarella
- ½ cup chicken breast, cooked and cubed

Method

1. Place a frying pan over medium heat.
2. Butter the outside of each slice of bread.
3. Mix together the filling ingredients and place onto the bread. Ensure the butter is on the outside of the sandwich when assembling.
4. Place the sandwich in the pan and fry for 3 minutes on each side. The bread should be golden.

Quiche in Ham Cups

Cal 190	**Difficulty:** Easy **Preparation time:** 10 minutes **Cook time:** 20 minutes **Servings:** 6

Nutrition per serving (g)

Fat	Saturates	Carbs	Sugars	Fiber	Protein	Salt
8.5	5.1	11.8	1.6	1.6	9.5	0.3

Ingredients

- 6 slices ham, cold cut, rounded
- 1 small bell pepper, diced
- ½ cup spring onion, green tips only
- 4 eggs, beaten
- 2 tbsp rice flour
- 4 tbsp lactose-free milk, can be substituted with other approved milk
- Pinch of salt
- Pinch of pepper

Method

1. Preheat the oven to 350°F and line 6 muffin tins with the ham slices.
2. Mix together the flour and milk, whisking constantly.
3. Add in the eggs, salt, and pepper, mixing until smooth. Add the spring onion and bell pepper. Pour carefully into the ham cups.
4. Bake for 15-20 minutes. It's ready when the quiche is puffy and the ham is crispy.
5. Let cool for 10 minutes then use a knife to carefully lift the quiche out of the tins.

Savory Muffins

Cal 120 — VEGETARIAN

Difficulty: Easy
Preparation time: 20 minutes
Cook time: 25 minutes
Servings: 12

Nutrition per serving (g)

Fat	Saturates	Carbs	Sugars	Fiber	Protein	Salt
4	0.8	15	0.5	1.5	4.9	0.3

Ingredients

- ¼ cup quinoa, boiled in ½ cup water
- 1 cup oat flour
- ¼ cup corn flour
- ¼ tsp cinnamon
- Pinch of salt
- Pinch of pepper
- 3 eggs
- ½ cup lactose-free or Greek yogurt
- 2 cups zucchini, grated
- ⅓ cup baby spinach, chopped
- A few sprigs of rosemary
- ¼ cup walnuts, chopped
- ½ lemon, zested

Method

1. Preheat the oven to 350°F and grease a 12-hole muffin pan.
2. In a saucepan, cook the quinoa in water for 15 minutes, then drain the excess water and let cool.
3. In a bowl, mix the dry ingredients together.
4. In a larger bowl, whisk the eggs and yogurt together, then add in the zucchini, spinach, nuts, spices, lemon zest, and quinoa slowly.
5. Add the bowl of dry ingredients to the larger bowl and mix well. Spoon the batter into muffin tins and bake for 25 minutes.

Feta, Chicken, and Pepper Sandwich

Cal 601

Difficulty: Easy
Preparation time: 5 minutes
Cook time: 20 minutes
Servings: 2

Nutrition per serving (g)

Fat	Saturates	Carbs	Sugars	Fiber	Protein	Salt
27	12.5	40	4	6	46	0.3

Ingredients

- 1 chicken breast fillet
- 1 tsp olive oil
- 4 slices gluten-free or spelt sourdough bread
- 1 cup feta cheese
- 1 large red capsicum, deseeded and cut into strips
- ¼ cup basil

Method

1. Cut the chicken in half to create thin fillets, drizzle olive oil over them, and season with salt and pepper. Place into a frying pan that has been heated over medium heat. Cook the fillets for 3 minutes on each side. Remove and cover with foil for 5 minutes before cutting into strips

2. Drizzle some oil onto one side of each slice of bread.

3. Assemble the sandwich by placing the feta, chicken, pepper, and basil, divided onto two slices of bread with the oil side down. Top with the other two slices of bread with the oil side facing up.

4. Cook the sandwiches in a frying pan for 3 minutes on each side until the bread is golden.

5. Remove from heat and serve.

Rice & Zucchini Slice

Cal 201 — VEGETARIAN

Difficulty: Medium
Preparation time: 5 minutes
Cook time: 55 minutes
Servings: 4

Nutrition per serving (g)

Fat	Saturates	Carbs	Sugars	Fiber	Protein	Salt
14	9.8	7.8	3.5	2	11.9	0.3

Ingredients

- ⅔ cup rice (brown, white, or basmati)
- ⅔ cup water
- 1 cup grated zucchini
- ½ cup grated carrot
- 3 eggs, beaten lightly
- 1 cup grated cheddar cheese

Method

1. Preheat the oven to 350°F. Line the base and sides of a loaf pan with parchment paper, leaving space for overhang.

2. Add rice and water to a saucepan and cook according to instructions on the packet.

3. In a bowl, add the zucchini, eggs, ½ cup cheese, rice, and carrot and mix well. Spread evenly over the bottom of the pan. Spread the remainder of the cheese over the top.

4. Bake for 30-35 minutes. When it's finished, the top should appear golden. Let cool before cutting into quarters. Place into a microwaveable, airtight Tupperware and put into the fridge within 2 hours of baking.

Cranberry Chocolate Chip Energy Bites

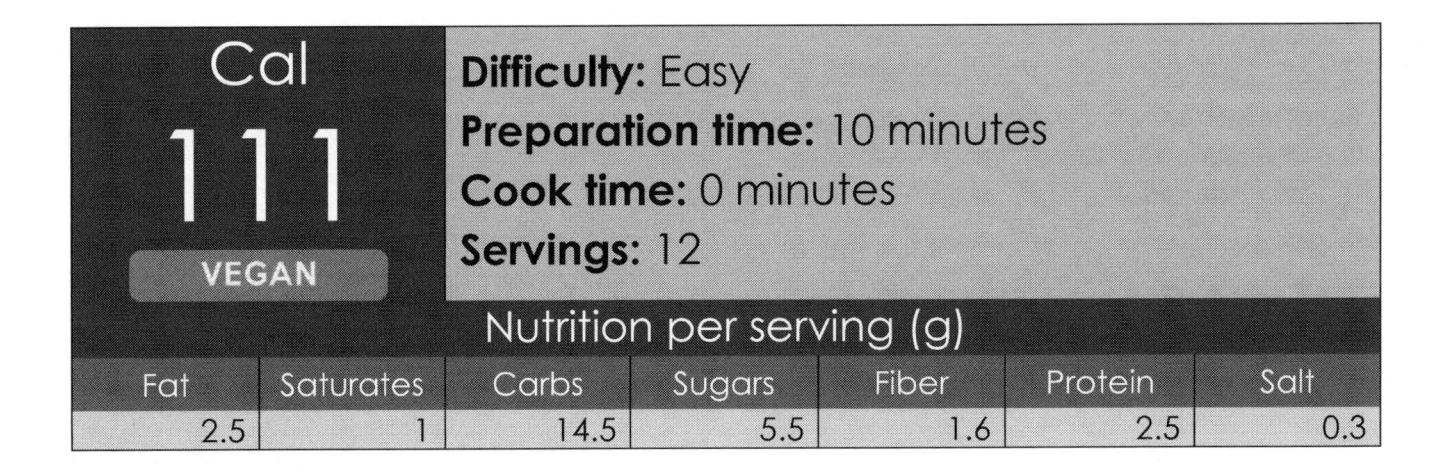

Cal 111 VEGAN

Difficulty: Easy
Preparation time: 10 minutes
Cook time: 0 minutes
Servings: 12

Nutrition per serving (g)

Fat	Saturates	Carbs	Sugars	Fiber	Protein	Salt
2.5	1	14.5	5.5	1.6	2.5	0.3

Ingredients

- ⅓ cup oats
- ½ cup cranberries, dried
- ⅓ cup peanut butter
- ¼ cup maple syrup
- 1 tbsp quinoa, puffed
- 2 tbsp mini dark chocolate chips

Method

1 Mix the oats in a blender or food processor until they are a flour-like consistency. Add the cranberries, peanut butter, and maple syrup, then blend until everything sticks together.

2 Add the quinoa and chocolate and mix until everything is evenly distributed.

3 Scoop a tablespoon at a time and roll into balls. Place in an airtight container and let rest in the fridge for at least 10 minutes. Store the remainder in the fridge until eaten.

4 It can be eaten for lunch or as a snack.

Cucumber salad

Cal 46.75
VEGETARIAN

Difficulty: Easy
Preparation time: 45 minutes
Cook time: -
Servings: 4

Nutrition per serving (g)

Fat	Saturates	Carbs	Sugars	Fiber	Protein	Salt
3	1.75	3.5	2.25	0.5	1.75	0.3

Ingredients

- ¾ cup cucumber
- 2 tbsp chives, fresh
- ½ cup Greek yogurt
- ¼ cup white vinegar

Method

1. Slice the cucumber thinly and place it into salad bowls along with the yogurt.

2. Chop the chives and mix them into the cucumber along with the vinegar.

3. Refrigerate until you are ready to eat.

Cheese, Ham, and Spinach Muffins

Cal 316

Difficulty: Easy
Preparation time: 10 minutes
Cook time: 20-25 minutes
Servings: 6

Nutrition per serving (g)

Fat	Saturates	Carbs	Sugars	Fiber	Protein	Salt
11.9	6	35.7	1.9	2.6	16.8	0.3

Ingredients

- 1 cup corn flour
- ¼ cup oats
- 2 ¼ tsp baking powder
- ½ tsp xanthan gum
- ½ cup thick Greek yogurt
- ⅔ cup lactose-free milk
- 2 large eggs
- 6 oz ham, lean
- ¼ cup chopped chives
- ½ cup cheddar cheese, grated (set 2 tbsp aside)
- ¼ cup baby spinach, chopped roughly
- ½ tsp paprika, smoked
- A drizzle of olive oil, used to grease the muffin tins

Method

1. Preheat the oven to 325°F and place a baking tray half-filled with water on the bottom shelf.

2. In a bowl, sift together the flour, baking powder, and xanthan gum, then stir in the oats.

3. In a smaller bowl, whisk the eggs, yogurt, and milk together, then add in the ham, chives, spinach, and cheese.

4. Make a well in the dry mix and pour the wet ingredients into it. Gently fold the ingredients together. The dough should be slightly wet but not liquid.

5. Grease the muffin tin and fill with the mixture. Wet your fingers and tap the top of the tin gently to settle the mixture.

6. Top with the remainder of the cheese and paprika.

7. Bake for 20-25 minutes.

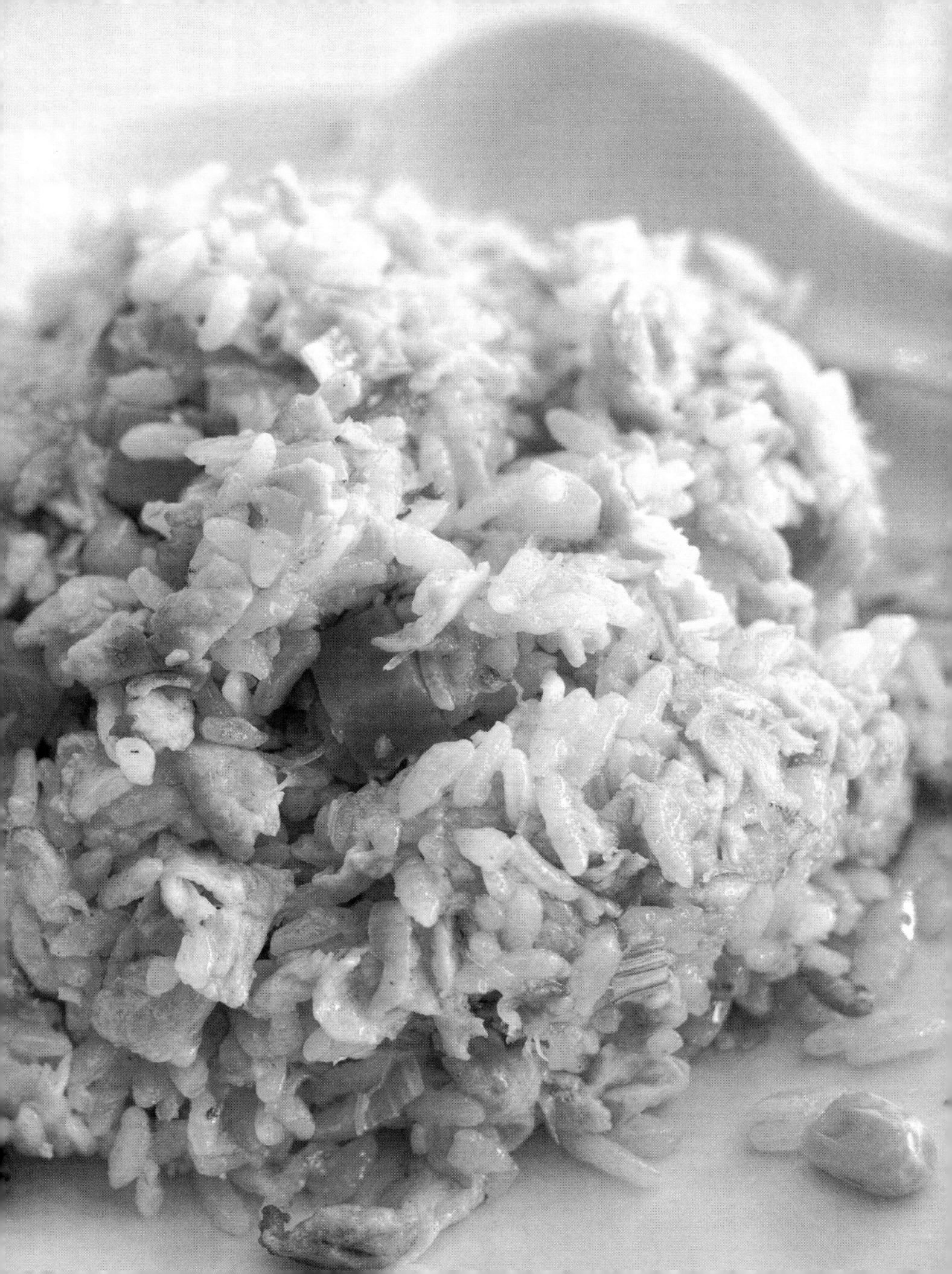

Dinner

Cheesy Chicken 84

Pork Tacos with Pineapple Salsa 85

Coconut Crusted Fish 86

Bolognese 88

Minestrone 89

Frittata `VEGETARIAN` 90

Tofu Skewers `VEGAN` 92

Baked Chicken Alfredo 94

Burgers 96

Day-Before Lamb Stew 98

Vegetable Fried Rice `VEGETARIAN` 99

Tuna, Bacon Quinoa Bowl 100

Roasted Pumpkin and Carrot Soup `VEGAN` 101

Feta Meatball 102

Spicy Tacos 103

Gnocchi `VEGETARIAN` 104

Vegan Curry `VEGAN` 106

Cheesy Chicken

Cal 661

Difficulty: Easy
Preparation time: 15 minutes
Cook time: 20 minutes
Servings: 4

Nutrition per serving (g)

Fat	Saturates	Carbs	Sugars	Fiber	Protein	Salt
35	11	14	14	2.5	71	0.3

Ingredients

- 4 chicken breasts, deboned and skinned
- 2 tsp olive oil
- 1 tbsp garlic-infused oil
- 1 celery stalk, no more than 2 inches, chopped finely
- 1 carrot, chopped finely
- 1 can (15 oz) tomatoes, chopped
- 3 tbsp tomato purée
- 1 ½ tsp oregano, dried
- ⅓ cup olives, pitted
- 6 slices mozzarella cheese

Method

1. Season the chicken with salt and pepper and set aside. Grease a deep-frying pan with oil and put over high heat. Cook the chicken in the pan for 3 minutes on each side. When each side is brown, transfer them to a plate.

2. Reduce the heat to low and add more oil. Add the vegetables and cook for 5 minutes. Stir while cooking. When the vegetables are soft, cook with garlic-infused oil for a few seconds.

3. Add the tomatoes, tinned and puréed, and stir in the oregano and olives. Bring to a boil for 5 minutes, stirring regularly. Reduce the heat.

4. Preheat the grill to its maximum.

5. Let the sauce simmer gently and add the chicken. Cook for 10 minutes and season to taste.

6. Put the mozzarella slices on top of the chicken and sauce, and sprinkle on black pepper. Place on the grill for 3 minutes, letting the cheese melt.

Pork Tacos with Pineapple Salsa

Cal 210

Difficulty: Easy
Preparation time: 10 minutes
Cook time: 15 minutes
Servings: 6 (1 taco per serving)

Nutrition per serving (g)

Fat	Saturates	Carbs	Sugars	Fiber	Protein	Salt
5.8	1.5	19.6	7	2	20	0.2

Ingredients

Pork
- 1 tbsp garlic-infused oil
- 1 spring onion, green part
- 1 jalapeño, optional
- 2 tbsp soy sauce
- 1 lb pork loin, boneless, cut into thin strips
- 2 tbsp sugar
- 2 tbsp water

Pineapple salsa
- 1 cup pineapple, chopped
- 1 cup cucumber, chopped
- ½ cup cilantro, chopped
- ½ cup spring onion, green part, chopped
- 1 tbsp lime juice
- Pinch of salt
- 6 corn tortillas

Method

1. In a heavy pan, heat the garlic-infused oil over medium heat. Add the spring onion and jalapeño (optional) and cook for 2 minutes. Turn the heat up and add the soy sauce and pork to the pan. Fry for a few minutes until the pork has no pink.

2. Add the sugar and water. Stir. Wait a minute. Stir and repeat until the pork is golden brown.

3. Prepare the salsa by mixing the ingredients together in a bowl.

4. Warm the tortillas in a skillet with oil. Spread the pork and salsa between the tortillas.

Coconut Crusted Fish

Cal 480

Difficulty: Medium
Preparation time: 15 minutes
Cook time: 30 minutes
Servings: 4

Nutrition per serving (g)

Fat	Saturates	Carbs	Sugars	Fiber	Protein	Salt
20	7.4	42.7	8.1	7.7	33	0.2

Ingredients

Coconut crust
- ¼ cup dried coconut, shredded
- 2 tbsp sesame oil
- ¼ cup spring onion, finely sliced, green part only
- 1 mild chili, green
- 4 lime leaves
- 1 lb white fish (haddock/cod/coley)
- ½ cup cheddar cheese, can substitute other approved cheeses

Chips
- 5 potatoes, approximately 1 ½ lbs, sliced
- Pinch of salt
- Pinch of pepper
- 1 tbsp sunflower oil

Salad
- 1 small cucumber, peeled
- 4 cups lettuce, shredded
- ½ red bell pepper, deseeded and sliced
- 4 medium tomatoes, cut into wedges
- 1 lemon

Method

1. In a bowl, place the shredded coconut and cover with water. Leave to soak for 10 minutes and then drain the water.

2. Prepare the vegetables.

3. Pour half the sesame oil in a pan over medium heat. Fry the chili, spring onion, and lime leaves until they look caramelized. Add the coconut and fry for a minute more. Set aside in a bowl.

4. Put the remainder of the oil and half the potatoes into the pan. Fry until golden and cooked. Repeat with the rest of the potatoes. Season to taste.

5. To prepare the salad, wash, chop, and mix the ingredients together. Squeeze the lemon juice over top.

6. Turn the oven onto the grill function to heat up.

7. Grease a medium pan with oil and cook the fish for 2 minutes on each side. Move the fish to a baking tray and top with cheese and coconut crust. Grill for 2 minutes. The crust should be golden when ready.

Bolognese

Cal 642

Difficulty: Easy
Preparation time: 5 minutes
Cook time: 40 minutes
Servings: 4

Nutrition per serving (g)

Fat	Saturates	Carbs	Sugars	Fiber	Protein	Salt
19	7.3	39.7	11	14.7	39.7	0.5

Ingredients

- 1 tbsp olive oil
- 1 lb ground beef, lean
- ½ cup leeks, tips only
- 1 can (14 oz) tomatoes, crushed
- 3 tbsp tomato paste
- 1 tsp oregano, dried
- 1 tsp thyme, dried
- 4 cups baby spinach
- Pinch of salt
- Pinch of pepper
- 1 ½ cups gluten-free spaghetti
- ½ cup approved cheese, grated
- 2 large carrots, peeled and cut into sticks
- ⅔ cup green beans

Method

1. Chop the spinach and leeks. Peel the carrots and cut into sticks. Slice the green beans. Put to one side.

2. Place a large pan over medium heat with olive oil in it. Cook the ground beef until it is browned. Add the tomatoes, leeks, spinach, and herbs to the beef. Mix well and let simmer for 20 minutes. Stir occasionally to ensure it does not burn. Season to taste.

3. In a large pot, add water and a generous amount of salt. Bring to a boil and add the spaghetti. Cook according to the packet instructions. Once cooked, drain and toss with olive oil.

4. Cook the green beans and carrots in a medium pot filled with boiling water for 2-3 minutes.

5. Serve the Bolognese on top of the spaghetti. Sprinkle with cheese and add the vegetables on the side.

Minestrone

Cal 386

Difficulty: Easy
Preparation time: 10 minutes
Cook time: 40 minutes
Servings: 4

Nutrition per serving (g)

Fat	Saturates	Carbs	Sugars	Fiber	Protein	Salt
17	3.9	50	11.8	10.6	11.9	1.1

Ingredients

- 3 oz bacon, optional
- 1 cup leeks, green parts
- 2 carrots, large
- 1 small potato
- ¼ cup celery, no more than 2 inches of stalk
- 1 tbsp garlic-infused oil
- 1 tsp olive oil
- 2 cups spinach
- ¾ cup zucchini
- 2 cans (15 oz each) of tomato, crushed
- 2 cups vegetable stock, no garlic or onion
- 1 ¼ cups boiling water
- ½ cup basil, fresh
- ½ cup gluten-free pasta, spirals or shells
- 1 cup chickpeas, in brine, drained
- 2 tbsp Parmesan, optional

Method

1. Dice the potato and carrots. Slice the celery and leeks. Remove the rind off the bacon before dicing. Add the garlic-infused oil, carrots, bacon, potatoes, celery, and leeks to a pan and sauté over medium heat for 15-20 minutes. These vegetables should be soft but not brown.

2. Dice the zucchini and slice the spinach. Make the stock by following the instructions on the packaging. Drain and rinse the chickpeas.

3. Add the tomatoes, stock, hot water, zucchini, spinach, and chickpeas to the pot. Summer for 10 minutes over medium heat.

4. Add the pasta and basil to the soup, setting aside a little basil for a garnish. Cook the pasta according to the instructions on the packet, using the soup as the water.

5. Season and garnish with basil and Parmesan.

Frittata

Cal **519** VEGETARIAN	**Difficulty:** Easy **Preparation time:** 30 minutes **Cook time:** 25 minutes **Servings:** 4

Nutrition per serving (g)

Fat	Saturates	Carbs	Sugars	Fiber	Protein	Salt
27	11.8	45	11	8.3	25	0.9

Ingredients

Roast vegetables
- 2 medium sweet potatoes, cubed
- 4 large carrots, cubed
- 1 tbsp olive oil

Frittata
- 6 large eggs
- ½ cup lactose-free milk, can be substituted with coconut or almond milk
- 1 tsp thyme, dried
- Pinch of salt
- Pinch of pepper
- ½ cup spring onions, green part, thinly sliced
- 1 bell pepper, finely diced
- 1 cup broccoli, cut into florets
- 1 cup green beans
- ¾ cup cheddar cheese, can substitute other approved cheeses

Tomato relish
- ½ tbsp garlic-infused oil
- 1 cup leeks, green leaves only, sliced finely
- 2 large tomatoes, diced
- 2 tbsp tomato paste
- 1 tbsp red wine vinegar
- 1 tbsp white sugar
- 1 tbsp brown sugar
- Pinch of paprika, smoked
- Pinch of salt
- Pinch of pepper

Method

1. Preheat the oven to 425°F. Line a roasting tray with parchment paper. Place the sweet potatoes and carrots on the tray. Toss with oil and season to taste. Roast for 20 minutes until tender.

2. In a small pan over medium heat, fry the leek leaves in garlic-infused oil for 2 minutes. Add the other relish ingredients and let the mixture simmer for 15 minutes. It should reduce and thicken.

3. To make the frittata, whisk the eggs and milk together until smooth. If using feta crumble, put it into the egg along with the herbs.

4. Fry the spring onion and pepper in an ovenproof pan over medium heat for 2 minutes. Remove from the heat and mix with the vegetables. Pour the egg over the vegetables and top with cheese.

5. Bake in the oven for 20 minutes. It should have a golden appearance. Allow to stand for 5 minutes and serve with the relish.

Tofu Skewers

Cal 523 VEGAN

Difficulty: Easy
Preparation time: 10 minutes (plus marinating overnight)
Cook time: 30 minutes
Servings: 4

Nutrition per serving (g)

Fat	Saturates	Carbs	Sugars	Fiber	Protein	Salt
15.9	2.2	70	9.8	5	25	1

Ingredients

Skewers

- 2 tbsp miso paste
- 1 tbsp garlic-infused oil
- 2 tbsp soy sauce
- ½ tsp crushed chili
- 1 ½ tbsp maple syrup
- 2 ½ cups (⅓ lb) tofu, firm, cubed
- 3 tsp sesame seeds for serving

Rice

- 1 ¼ cup basmati rice

Salad

- 3 cups lettuce
- 1 small cucumber, peeled and cut into chunks
- 1 cup spring onion, green tips, sliced finely
- 1 ⅓ cups green beans, cut in pieces
- 1 tbsp olive oil
- Juice from half an orange
- Pinch of salt
- Pinch of pepper

Method

1. Mix together the miso paste, garlic oil, soy sauce, chili, and maple syrup in a small bowl. Cover the tofu with half the marinade and soak overnight.

2. Preheat the oven to 375°F.

3. Cook the rice according to the instructions on the packet.

4. Prepare the salad by peeling and cutting the cucumber. Boil the green beans until bright green and then drain and rinse in cold water. Slice the spring onion tips. Toss the salad in a bowl with a drizzle of olive oil, orange juice, salt, and pepper.

5. On four skewers, divide the tofu. Bake in the oven for 12 minutes. When finished, the tofu should look caramelized.

6. Heat the remaining half of the marinade. Serve the skewers hot with sesame seeds used as a garnish and the rice and salad. Drizzle the remainder of the miso over the dish.

Baked Chicken Alfredo

Cal 743	**Difficulty:** Easy **Preparation time:** 35 minutes **Cook time:** 15 minutes **Servings:** 4 large servings

Nutrition per serving (g)

Fat	Saturates	Carbs	Sugars	Fiber	Protein	Salt
29	9	78.8	11	10	41	0.6

Ingredients

Pasta and chicken

- ½ lb chicken breast fillets, cut into chunks
- 1 tsp olive oil
- Pinch of salt
- Pinch of pepper
- 1 cup gluten-free pasta
- 4 cups baby spinach, chopped roughly
- 2 cups broccoli, florets
- ½ cup spring onion, green part
- ½ cup cheddar cheese
- 2 tbsp sage, fresh, chopped finely

Sauce

- 4 tbsp butter
- ¼ cup gluten-free flour
- 3 cups lactose-free milk
- ½ cup cheddar cheese
- 2 tbsp Parmesan, grated (optional)
- ½ tsp basil, dried
- Pinch of salt
- Pinch of pepper

Method

1. Preheat the oven to 350°F. Grease a large oven dish. Place a pot of water over medium heat to boil for the pasta.

2. Prepare the chicken by rubbing salt and pepper on it and then cutting into chunks. Chop the spinach, cut the broccoli, slice the spring onion, and grate the cheese.

3. Over medium heat, sear the chicken in a pan with oil and place to the side. Place the spinach in the pan and cook until slightly wilted, about 1 minute. Set to the side.

4. While the chicken cooks, place a saucepan over medium heat and melt the butter. Whisk in the flour. Cook for 1 minute, stirring continuously.

5. Whisk in ½ cup of milk. When smooth, whisk in the remainder of the milk a cup at a time. Season with salt, pepper, basil, and half the Parmesan. Stir occasionally and allow the sauce to thicken.

6. Cook the pasta for 5 minutes, then drain and toss with olive oil. Mix the pasta with the chicken, sauce, and vegetables. Transfer it into the oven dish, top with cheese, and bake for 10 minutes uncovered. Remove the lid of the dish and grill for 3 minutes and top with sage.

Burgers

Cal 613	**Difficulty:** Easy **Preparation time:** 15 minutes **Cook time:** 30 minutes **Servings:** 4

Nutrition per serving (g)

Fat	Saturates	Carbs	Sugars	Fiber	Protein	Salt
22	5.6	62	19.6	12.7	39.9	0.9

Ingredients

Patties

- ½ lb ground beef, lean
- ¼ cup spring onion, green part, chopped finely
- ¼ cup gluten-free breadcrumbs (can be crumbled bread slices)
- 1 egg
- ½ tsp thyme, dried
- 1 tsp oregano, dried
- 1 tsp basil, dried
- 1 tbsp Worcestershire sauce
- Pinch of salt
- Pinch of pepper

Side salad

- 3 large carrots, peeled and cut into chunks
- 1 ½ tsp sunflower oil
- Pinch of salt
- Pinch of pepper
- 4 cups lettuce
- 1 cucumber, small
- 3 tomatoes, medium

Garnish

- 4 tbsp approved sauce, from the approved list
- 4 gluten-free buns

Method

1. Preheat the oven to 400°F. Place the peeled and cut carrots on a roasting tray with oil. Bake for 25-30 minutes, turning halfway through

2. To make the patties, first, whisk the egg in a small bowl. In a large bowl, mix the ground beef, spring onion, breadcrumbs, herbs, Worcestershire sauce, egg, salt, and pepper. Divide the mixture evenly into patties.

3. Fry the patties over medium heat for 7 minutes on each side.

4. Prepare the salad by washing and shredding the lettuce and chopping the tomatoes and cucumber.

5. Assemble the burger by placing the patties onto rolls. On the side, place the carrots and salad. Add an approved sauce onto the burger if desired.

Day-Before Lamb Stew

Cal 703

Difficulty: Difficult
Preparation time: 20 minutes
Cook time: 10 hours
Servings: 4

Nutrition per serving (g)

Fat	Saturates	Carbs	Sugars	Fiber	Protein	Salt
35.8	12.8	64	12	9	33.4	1.5

Ingredients

- ½ lb lamb, deboned
- 1 tbsp sunflower oil
- 1 ½ cups leeks, green tips
- 2 carrots, large
- 1 ½ cups pumpkin or sweet potato, cubed
- 3 cups potatoes, cubed
- 4 cups vegetable stock, no garlic or onion
- 1 cup boiling water
- 1 tsp oregano, dried
- ½ tsp thyme, dried
- Pinch of salt
- Pinch of pepper
- 1 cup green beans
- 3 tbsp parsley, fresh for garnish
- 8 slices gluten-free bread

Method

1. Use a slow cooker with cooking oil on low. Remove the fat from the lamb and cut into cubes.

2. In a frying pan over medium heat, brown the lamb for 5 minutes. Add the lamb to the slow cooker.

3. Clean the vegetables, peeling the sweet potato, carrots, and potato, then cutting them into cubes. Add to the slow cooker.

4. Add the garlic-infused oil, herbs, and heated vegetable stock into the slow cooker. Next, add the boiling water and season with pepper.

5. Cook the stew on low for 10 hours. Check the meat after 10 hours, and if it is soft, break the meat up softly with a fork to help it thicken.

6. Trim the green beans and place them into boiling water for 3 minutes before stirring into the stew. It is ready to be served.

7. Toast the bread and serve with a bowl of stew.

Vegetable Fried Rice

Cal 310
VEGETARIAN

Difficulty: Easy
Preparation time: 5 minutes
Cook time: 15 minutes
Servings: 2

Nutrition per serving (g)

Fat	Saturates	Carbs	Sugars	Fiber	Protein	Salt
17.1	5.8	28.2	4.3	2.1	10.7	0.5

Ingredients

- 1 ½ cups rice, cooked and cooled
- 1 ½ tsp garlic-infused oil
- 2 eggs, whisked
- 2 carrots, chopped finely
- 2 cups vegetables (zucchini, bell peppers, and leeks), chopped into cubes
- 4 spring onions, green parts
- Pinch of salt
- 1 tbsp ginger, minced
- 2 tbsp sesame oil
- 1 tbsp soy sauce
- 1 tsp chili flakes, crushed

Method

1. In a large pan over medium heat, heat 1 tablespoon of garlic-infused oil. Add the egg, and cook until scrambled, stirring occasionally. Transfer the egg to another plate.

2. Heat the remaining ½ teaspoon of oil over medium heat, then add the carrots and other vegetables. Cook for 8 minutes until the carrot is soft.

3. Add the rice, onion, ginger, salt, and soy sauce to the pan. Stir for 3 minutes, then mix the egg into the dish.

4. Remove from the heat and stir in the sesame oil and chili flakes before serving.

Tuna, Bacon Quinoa Bowl

Cal 288

Difficulty: Easy
Preparation time: 20 minutes
Cook time: 10 minutes
Servings: 2

Nutrition per serving (g)

Fat	Saturates	Carbs	Sugars	Fiber	Protein	Salt
6	1.5	34.5	1.5	3.5	22	0.3

Ingredients

Vinaigrette

- ½ cup olive oil
- 2 tbsp rice vinegar
- 2 tbsp lemon juice, fresh
- 1 tbsp Dijon mustard
- 1 tsp parsley, dried
- ½ tbsp garlic-infused oil
- Pinch of salt
- Pinch of pepper

Bowl

- 1 ½ cups quinoa, cooked
- ½ pack bacon
- 1 can (3 oz) of tuna, shredded, in brine
- 1 small cucumber, sliced
- ¼ cup cherry tomatoes, halved

Method

1. Combine the vinaigrette ingredients into a jar with an airtight lid. Shake well and let sit for 30 minutes before use.

2. Cook the quinoa according to the package instructions. Dice the bacon, and then fry it. Store all ingredients in separate containers.

3. Assemble each bowl by combining the ingredients and drizzling dressing over just before eating.

Roasted Pumpkin and Carrot Soup

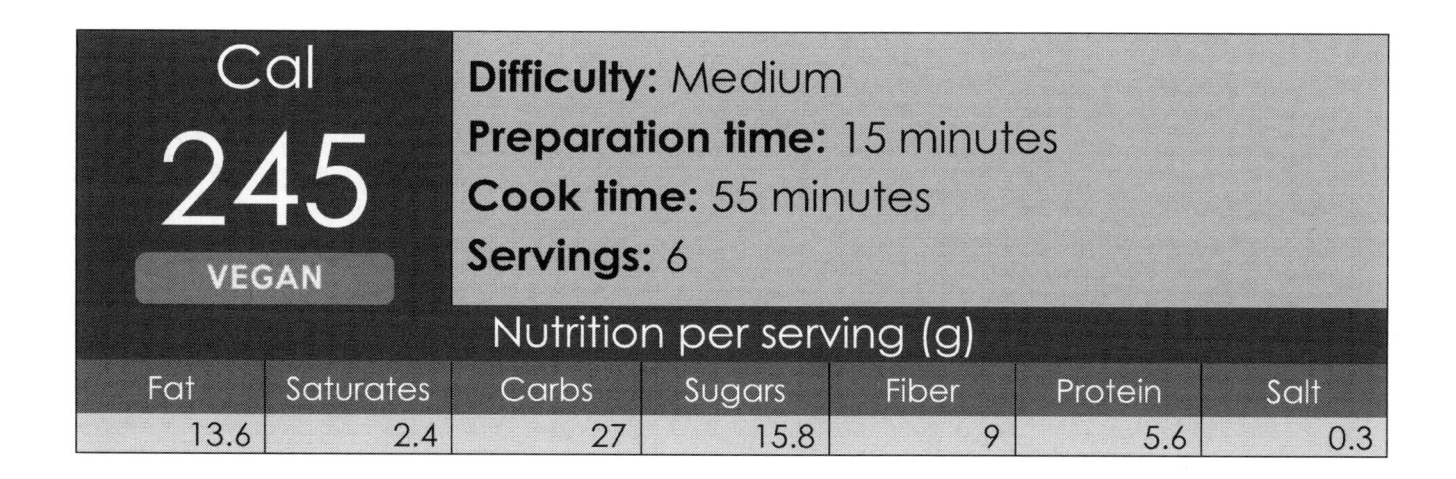

Cal 245
VEGAN

Difficulty: Medium
Preparation time: 15 minutes
Cook time: 55 minutes
Servings: 6

Nutrition per serving (g)

Fat	Saturates	Carbs	Sugars	Fiber	Protein	Salt
13.6	2.4	27	15.8	9	5.6	0.3

Ingredients

- 7 cups pumpkin, peeled and cubed
- 4 ½ cups carrots, peeled and cubed
- 3 tbsp olive oil
- 1 ½ tbsp garlic-infused oil
- 2 tsp coriander, ground
- 1 tsp cumin, ground
- 1 tsp turmeric, ground
- ½ tsp cardamom, ground
- ¼ tsp chili powder
- 4 ½ cups vegetable stock, no onion or garlic
- 2 ¼ cups water

Method

1. Preheat the oven to 400°F. On a lined tray, place the carrots and pumpkin and drizzle with oil. Bake for 35 minutes.

2. Heat the remainder of the oil in a pot, then add the seeds and spices. Allow them to cook until the mustard seeds pop.

3. Place all the ingredients into the pot and cook for 15 minutes.

4. Allow the mixture to cool for 15 minutes and then blend and serve.

Feta Meatball

Cal 619

Difficulty: Easy
Preparation time: 15 minutes
Cook time: 15 minutes
Servings: 1

Nutrition per serving (g)

Fat	Saturates	Carbs	Sugars	Fiber	Protein	Salt
44	12.5	9	2.7	2.9	44	0.3

Ingredients

- 1 lb lean ground beef
- ⅓ cup feta cheese
- 2 slices bread, crumbled
- 2 ½ tbsp parsley, chopped
- 1 ½ tbsp tomato paste
- 1 cup cherry tomatoes
- 1 lb pasta
- A drizzle of red wine vinegar
- ¼ cup kale, chopped
- 1 tbsp basil, firmly packed
- 2 tbsp roasted almonds
- 1 ½ tbsp garlic-infused oil
- 4 tbsp olive oil
- 2 ½ tbsp lemon juice
- 1 tbsp Parmesan cheese

Method

1. Preheat the oven to 425° F and line a baking tray with parchment paper.

2. First, make the pesto. Place the kale, basil, Parmesan, and almonds into a food processor and mix until finely chopped. Slowly add the oil and lemon in a thin stream. Once mixed, set aside.

3. In a bowl, mix the ground beef, feta, bread crumbs, tomato paste, and parsley. Once mixed together, roll the mixture into balls. Use about a tablespoon of mixture per ball. After rolling, place them onto the baking tray. Drizzle with a small amount of olive oil and bake for 10 minutes. Add the tomatoes and bake for 10 more minutes.

4. While the meatballs are in the oven, cook the pasta according to the instructions on the package. When draining, keep ⅓ of the pasta water. Add the pesto and pasta water to the pot with the pasta.

5. Serve with the meatballs, tomatoes, and a small amount of red wine vinegar.

Spicy Tacos

Cal 450

Difficulty: Easy
Preparation time: 20 minutes
Cook time: 10 minutes
Servings: 6

Nutrition per serving (g)

Fat	Saturates	Carbs	Sugars	Fiber	Protein	Salt
27	12	17	2.5	5	33	0.3

Ingredients

Seasoning
- 2 ½ tsp ground cumin
- 1 ½ tsp smoked paprika
- 1 tsp chili powder
- 1 tsp dried oregano
- ½ tsp black pepper

Filling
- 1 lb your choice of protein (chicken, fish, or ground beef)
- 2 tomatoes, diced
- 2 lettuce leaves, large
- 1 jalapeño
- 12 corn tortillas
- 1 cup shredded cheddar cheese
- 1 cup coriander, fresh and chopped
- Thick Greek yogurt

Method

1. Mix the seasoning ingredients together in a jar or bowl.

2. In a heated pan greased with oil, add the seasoning and stir for 30 seconds. Then, add the protein and cook thoroughly.

3. Fill the tortillas with the vegetables and protein. Top with coriander and yogurt and serve.

Gnocchi

Cal 504 VEGETARIAN	**Difficulty:** Medium **Preparation time:** 5 minutes **Cook time:** 20 minutes **Servings:** 2

Nutrition per serving (g)

Fat	Saturates	Carbs	Sugars	Fiber	Protein	Salt
19	3.8	65.9	4.5	4.9	13.5	0.3

Ingredients

- 2 tbsp blanched almonds, toasted and chopped
- 1 tbsp garlic-infused oil
- 2 tbsp olive oil
- 2 tbsp Parmesan
- ½ cup cherry tomatoes, cut in half
- ¼ cup green beans
- 1 lb gnocchi
- 1 lemon, juiced
- ¼ cup rocket
- Pepper to taste
- Salt to taste
- 1 tbsp olive oil

Method

1. In a pot, combine a pinch of salt and water, filling half the pot, and boil over high heat.

2. In a small bowl, add the almonds and a pinch of salt and pepper.

3. Mix the finely chopped basil with 1 tablespoon olive oil and 1 tablespoon garlic. Add to the bowl with the almonds and salt. Grate half the Parmesan into the bowl with salt and pepper.

4. Add the halved tomatoes to the mix, and use your hands to mix everything together.

5. Trim and boil the green beans in a small pot for 4 minutes. Once tender, cut into strips lengthwise.

6. Boil the gnocchi for 3 minutes in the pot of boiling water. When they are floating, they are ready. Drain them, but keep some of the water. In the same pan as the gnocchi and cooking water, add the pesto and beans. Cook on low heat and stir until the gnocchi is covered.

7. In a bowl, add one tablespoon of olive oil, salt, pepper, and lemon juice. Mix the rocket into the dressing.

8. Serve the gnocchi with the rocket and the remainder of the cheese on top.

Vegan Curry

Cal 471 VEGAN

Difficulty: Easy
Preparation time: 20 minutes
Cook time: 40 minutes
Servings: 4

Nutrition per serving (g)

Fat	Saturates	Carbs	Sugars	Fiber	Protein	Salt
29	11.9	38.9	12	8	8.4	0.5

Ingredients

- 1 ½ cups pumpkin or sweet potato
- 1 cup carrots
- 1 cup eggplant
- ½ bunch fresh coriander
- 1 cup canned chickpeas in water, rinsed
- 1 ½ tbsp olive oil
- ¼ tsp chili flakes
- 1 ½ tsp ground coriander
- 1 tsp ground turmeric
- 1 tsp ground cumin
- 2 tsp crushed ginger
- 2 tbsp garlic-infused oil
- ½ cup green tips of spring onions
- ½ cup coconut milk, canned
- 1 cup vegetable stock, no onion or garlic
- 1 dried bay leaf
- 1 ½ tbsp soy sauce
- 2 ½ tbsp tomato paste
- 1 lime, zest
- 1 tsp sugar
- 1 ½ cups cooked basmati rice
- 2 tbsp cornstarch

Method

1. Preheat the oven to 350°F. Place the chickpeas and eggplant on a lined tray. Cook for 10 minutes, then flip the eggplant and chickpeas and cook for another 10 minutes.

2. While the eggplant and chickpeas are in the oven, cook the rice according to the instructions on the packet.

3. In a large frying pan over medium heat, add the spices, garlic oil, and spring onion. Fry for two minutes.

4 Add the coconut milk, vegetable stock, soy sauce, bay leaf, and tomato paste to the pan. Mix well.

5 Add the pumpkin and carrots to the pan and bring to a simmer. Once it simmers, cover and cook on low heat for 20 minutes. Stir occasionally. Add small amounts of water if the mixture looks too dry.

6 When the vegetables are soft, add 2 tablespoons of cornstarch dissolved in warm water to the curry. The curry should thicken.

7 While it thickens, add the lime zest and sugar. Remove the bay leaf and fold the eggplant into the mix.

8 Serve the curry on top of rice with the fresh coriander and roasted chickpeas used as a garnish.

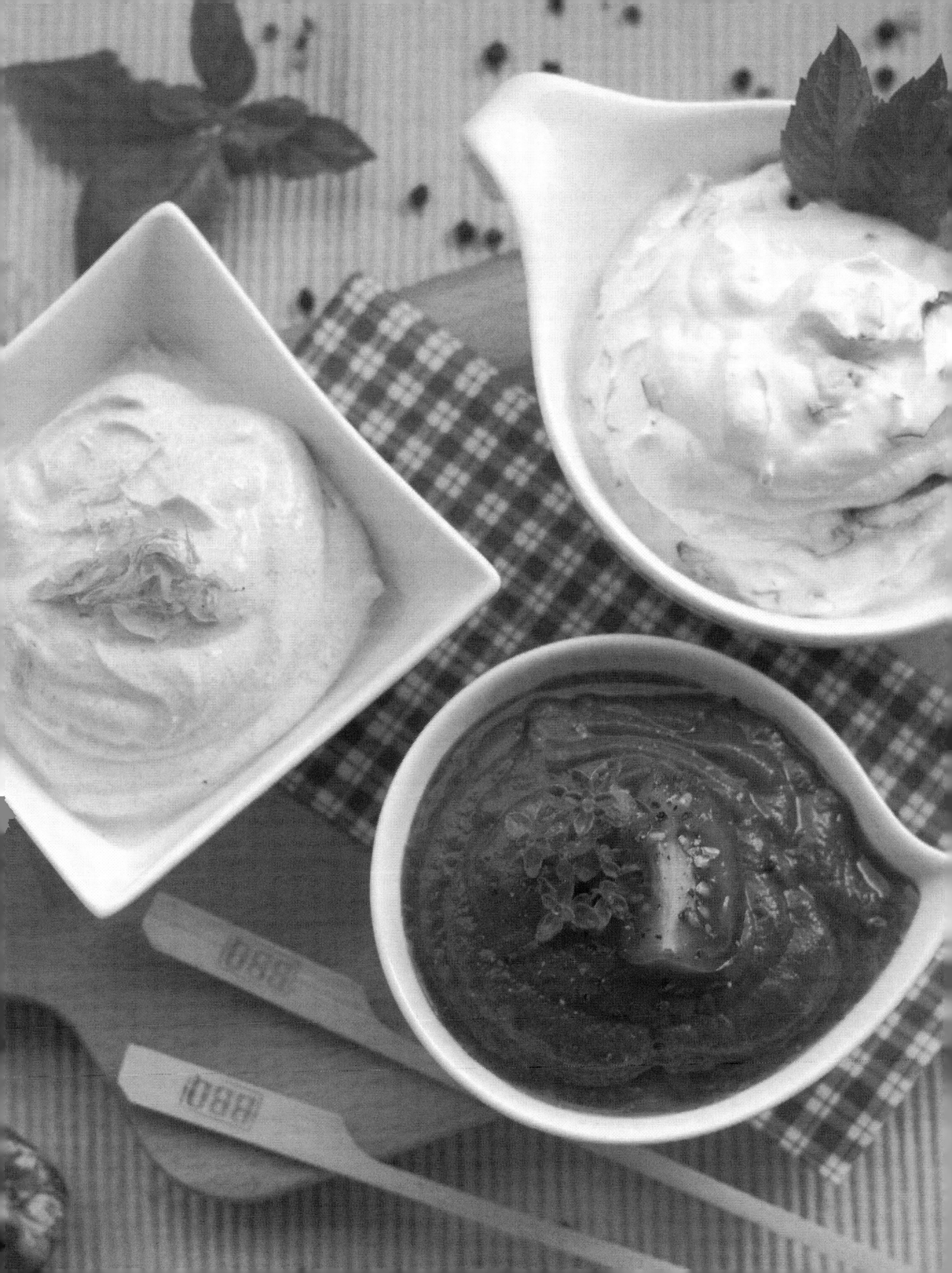

Side Dishes and Starters

Parmesan Mayo Corn on the Cob `VEGETARIAN` 110

Garden Medley `VEGAN` 111

Zucchini Fritters `VEGETARIAN` 112

Pumpkin Cornbread `VEGETARIAN` 113

Veggie Dip `VEGETARIAN` 114

Mashed Potatoes `VEGETARIAN` 115

Festive Stuffing `VEGAN` 116

Chicken Cheese Fritters 117

Rice Paper "Spring Rolls" with Satay Sauce `VEGAN` 118

Chive Dip `VEGAN` 120

Roast Vegetables `VEGAN` 121

Beetroot Dip `VEGAN` 122

Parmesan Mayo Corn on the Cob

Cal 254
VEGETARIAN

Difficulty: Easy
Preparation time: 5 minutes
Cook time: 10 minutes
Servings: 6

Nutrition per serving (g)

Fat	Saturates	Carbs	Sugars	Fiber	Protein	Salt
15	5.8	20	3.8	1.8	12.8	0.2

Ingredients

- 6 ears of corn, leaves still attached
- ½ cup mayonnaise
- ⅔ cup grated Parmesan
- 1 tbsp coriander, chopped

Method

1. In a pot of salted, boiling water, cook the corn for 7 minutes before draining. Leave to cool. Once cooled, pull back the leaves and place the corn onto a hot, greased skillet and grill for 5 minutes making sure to roll them until there are char marks.

2. In a bowl, mix the mayonnaise, Parmesan, and coriander. When the corn is ready, spread a tablespoon of the mayonnaise mixture onto each cob.

3. Serve warm.

Garden Medley

Cal 149

VEGAN

Difficulty: Easy
Preparation time: 5 minutes
Cook time: 25 minutes
Servings: 6

Nutrition per serving (g)

Fat	Saturates	Carbs	Sugars	Fiber	Protein	Salt
11	6	10.5	12	2	2	0.5

Ingredients

- ¾ cup water
- 4 carrots, cut into strips
- ¼ cup butter or margarine
- 1 yellow squash, cut lengthwise
- 3 tbsp green pepper, chopped
- 1 tbsp chopped basil
- Pinch of salt

Method

1. In a pot, bring the water to a boil and add the carrots. Cover the pot and let cook for 8-10 minutes.

2. Drain the water from the pot and add the butter to melt, stirring to keep the butter from burning. Add the pepper, basil, and salt to the pot and mix well.

3. Place the squash into the pot and cook covered for 8 minutes. The squash should be crispy but still tender.

4. Once the vegetables are tender, serve on a plate.

Zucchini Fritters

Cal 310
VEGETARIAN

Difficulty: Easy
Preparation time: 10 minutes
Cook time: 15 minutes
Servings: 3 (2-3 fritters per serving)

Nutrition per serving (g)

Fat	Saturates	Carbs	Sugars	Fiber	Protein	Salt
17.2	5.8	28.2	4.3	2.1	10.7	0.5

Ingredients

Fritters

- 2 cups broccoli, cut into florets
- ¼ cup zucchini, grated
- ½ cup cheddar cheese, grated (other approved cheeses can be substituted)
- Pinch of salt
- Pinch of pepper
- 1 egg
- ½ cup gluten-free flour
- 3 tbsp lactose-free milk, can be substituted with other approved milk
- 1 tbsp garlic-infused oil

Lime aioli

- ¼ cup mayonnaise
- 2 tsp lime juice, fresh
- ½ tsp lime zest

Method

1. Cut the broccoli, steam it, then mash it. Grate the zucchini.

2. In a bowl, mix the wet ingredients. Add the dry ingredients, excluding the black pepper, into the bowl, then fold in the broccoli, zucchini, and cheese. Do not over mix.

3. Over medium heat, place a large pan that has been greased lightly with oil. With a ¼-cup measuring spoon, scoop some mixture and pour it into the pan then flatten gently with a spatula. Cook 2-3 fritters per batch.

4. Whisk the lime juice, zest, and mayonnaise and season with black pepper.

5. Serve the fritters topped with the aioli.

Pumpkin Cornbread

Cal 230
VEGETARIAN

Difficulty: Medium
Preparation time: 10 minutes
Cook time: 25 minutes
Servings: 8

Nutrition per serving (g)

Fat	Saturates	Carbs	Sugars	Fiber	Protein	Salt
5.8	1.1	39.5	9.8	2	4.9	0.6

Ingredients

- 1 ¼ cups corn flour
- 1 cup gluten-free, all-purpose flour
- 2 tsp of baking powder
- ¾ tsp of baking soda
- 1 tbsp white sugar
- 1 tbsp brown sugar
- Pinch of salt
- 1 ½ tsp sage, dried
- ½ cup spring onions, green part only
- 1 cup cheese, cheddar or any other approved
- 1 cup pumpkin, puréed
- 1 cup lactose-free milk
- 2 tbsp olive oil

Method

1. Preheat the oven to 350°F.
2. Chop the spring onions finely and grate the cheese.
3. Mix the flour, baking powder, baking soda, sugar, salt, and sage together in a bowl.
4. Melt the butter and use it to grease an ovenproof skillet. Once greased, add the remainder of the butter in the bowl.
5. Mix all the ingredients together thoroughly, then scoop and spread the mixture into the skillet.
6. Bake for 30-35 minutes. When finished, the top should be golden. Insert a skewer into the middle of the pan, and if it comes out clean, the bread is fully cooked.

Veggie Dip

Cal 123 — VEGETARIAN

Difficulty: Easy
Preparation time: 5 minutes
Cook time: 5 minutes
Servings: 16

Nutrition per serving (g)

Fat	Saturates	Carbs	Sugars	Fiber	Protein	Salt
10	1	3	1	3	3	0.3

Ingredients

- 1 cup mayonnaise
- 2 cups Greek yogurt
- 2 cups kale, chopped finely
- 1 ½ cups bell peppers, variety of colors, chopped finely
- 2 cups water chestnuts, chopped finely
- 3 spring onions, green parts only, chopped finely
- 1 tsp garlic-infused oil
- Pinch of salt
- Fresh sliced vegetables and corn chips for serving

Method

1. In a bowl, mix all the ingredients well, except for the fresh sliced vegetables. Place in the fridge until serving.
2. Serve with the fresh vegetables.

Mashed Potatoes

Cal 106 — VEGETARIAN

Difficulty: Easy
Preparation time: 15 minutes
Cook time: 15 minutes
Servings: 14 (½ cup each)

Nutrition per serving (g)

Fat	Saturates	Carbs	Sugars	Fiber	Protein	Salt
5	2	11	2	4	3	0.2

Ingredients

- 4 large Russet potatoes
- 1 tbsp rosemary, fresh, chopped
- 2 tbsp butter or margarine
- 2 tbsp olive oil
- ½ cup feta cheese
- ½ cup lactose-free milk
- Pinch of salt

Method

1. Wash and peel the potatoes, then cut into cubes. Place them into a pot and cover with water. Add a little extra water to allow for evaporation. Cover the pot and bring the water to a boil, then lower the heat, remove the lid, and cook until the potatoes feel tender when poked with a fork. Carefully pour out the water and leave open for 5 minutes.

2. While the potatoes are cooking, chop the rosemary.

3. After the five minutes, add the ingredients, except the salt and rosemary, to the pot and mash the ingredients together until you reach the desired consistency. Add rosemary and salt to taste.

Festive Stuffing

Cal 120
VEGAN

Difficulty: Medium
Preparation time: 10 minutes
Cook time: 20 minutes
Servings: 12 (small)

Nutrition per serving (g)

Fat	Saturates	Carbs	Sugars	Fiber	Protein	Salt
5.6	0.9	14.8	1.6	0.9	3	0.3

Ingredients

- 10 slices gluten-free bread, can use other approved bread
- 4 tbsp butter or margarine
- 1 tsp garlic-infused oil
- 1 ½ cups leeks, only the green tips
- ½ cup parsley, fresh
- 1 tsp sage, dried
- 1 tsp oregano, dried
- ½ tsp thyme, dried
- Pinch of salt
- Pinch of pepper
- ½ cup vegetable stock, low-FODMAP-approved, without onion or garlic

Method

1. Preheat the oven to 350°F.

2. In a large bowl, tear the bread into small pieces.

3. In a smaller bowl, melt the butter and mix the garlic-infused oil into it before drizzling and tossing it onto the bread. Spread the bread over an oven tray, then place it in the oven for 5 minutes. Toss the bread and bake for another 5 minutes.

4. Depending on the desired texture, place the bread and other ingredients into a bowl for a chunky texture or a blender for a smooth texture. Mix well.

5. Grease a muffin tin with oil. Mix the stock into the bread, being careful not to make the bread soggy. Spoon the mixture into the muffin tin, fill each space to the top, and press down gently.

6. Bake for 10-15 minutes. When finished, the top should be crunchy.

Chicken Cheese Fritters

Cal 415

Difficulty: Easy
Preparation time: 5 minutes
Cook time: 20 minutes
Servings: 4 (3 fritters per serving)

Nutrition per serving (g)

Fat	Saturates	Carbs	Sugars	Fiber	Protein	Salt
26.8	8	11.4	1.7	0.4	31.5	0.7

Ingredients

Fritters
- 1 lb ground chicken
- 2 eggs, large
- ¼ cup mayonnaise
- ¼ cup gluten-free, all-purpose flour
- ¾ cup mozzarella cheese, grated
- 2 tbsp basil, fresh and finely chopped
- 2 tbsp chives, dried
- Pinch of salt
- Pinch black pepper
- 1 tsp sunflower oil

Aioli
- ¼ cup mayonnaise
- ¼ tsp garlic-infused oil
- ½ tbsp lemon juice
- 1 tsp lemon zest
- Pinch of salt
- Pinch of black pepper

Method

1. In a bowl, mix the chicken with the fritter ingredients. Mix until combined thoroughly.

2. Over medium heat, place a pan greased with oil. When the oil is hot, measure a ¼ cup of the fritter mixture and pour it into the pan and flatten with a spatula.

3. Fry for 3-4 minutes until the fritters are golden brown. Add oil if needed. Place the cooked fritters onto a paper towel to absorb the oil.

4. The aioli is made by mixing the ingredients in a small bowl until smooth.

5. Serve the fritters with aioli on the side.

Rice Paper "Spring Rolls" with Satay Sauce

Cal 472
VEGAN

Difficulty: Medium
Preparation time: 20 minutes
Cook time: 30 minutes
Servings: 3 (4 rolls per serving)

Nutrition per serving (g)

Fat	Saturates	Carbs	Sugars	Fiber	Protein	Salt
23.5	4.7	48.2	17	3.7	24.4	0.9

Ingredients

Satay sauce

- 4 tbsp peanut butter
- 2 tbsp lemon juice
- 2 tbsp water
- 2 tsp brown sugar
- 1 tsp white sugar

Rice spring rolls

- 12 rice paper wrappers
- 1 cucumber, small
- 1 carrot, large, cut into matchstick pieces
- 1 cup red cabbage, sliced finely
- ½ cup mint, fresh, chopped roughly
- ½ cup cilantro, fresh, roughly cut

Method

1. Prepare the satay sauce first. Soften the peanut butter in a microwaveable bowl for about 30 seconds. Place the rest of the sauce ingredients into the bowl and use a fork to mix until smooth. Add a tbsp of water if the mixture is too thick.

2. Put warm water into a large bowl. One at a time, dip a rice wrapper into the water until it softens slightly then place it on a clean, damp cloth.

3. Place a small amount of the fresh vegetables and herbs onto the bottom third of the wrapper. Do not overfill as it will affect the rolling process.

4 To roll, first, fold the small sides up like a burrito. Next, pull the bottom of the wrapper up gently over the filling. It is best to hold the end with the filling in it in your hands.

5 The rolls are best when dipped in the satay sauce.

Chive Dip

Cal 82 VEGAN

Difficulty: Easy
Preparation time: 5 minutes
Cook time: 30 minutes
Servings: 10

Nutrition per serving (g)

Fat	Saturates	Carbs	Sugars	Fiber	Protein	Salt
7.8	1.2	2.9	0.8	0.3	0.4	0.2

Ingredients

- 2 tbsp parsley, fresh, chopped finely
- 1 cup mayonnaise
- 2 tbsp chives, dried
- 2 tbsp oil (best with onion-infused but can be substituted with other approved oils)
- Pinch of salt
- 1 tsp lemon juice

Method

1. Mix the mayonnaise, oil, chives, salt, and parsley together in a bowl. Add lemon juice or herbs of choice to taste.

2. Chill in the fridge for 30 minutes and serve with approved fresh vegetables or chips.

Roast Vegetables

Cal 316 VEGAN

Difficulty: Easy
Preparation time: 15 minutes
Cook time: 45 minutes
Servings: 6

Nutrition per serving (g)

Fat	Saturates	Carbs	Sugars	Fiber	Protein	Salt
10.2	1.5	52.9	15.8	10.3	6.1	0.2

Ingredients

Vegetables
- 1 ½ cups carrot
- 1 ½ cups parsnip
- 1 ½ cups pumpkin
- 2 red bell peppers
- 1 ¾ cup potatoes
- 1 ⅓ cup baby beetroot, drained
- Pinch of salt
- Pinch of pepper

Glaze
- 4 tbsp olive oil
- 1 ½ tbsp ginger, crushed
- 1 tbsp maple syrup

Method

1. Preheat the oven to 375ºF and line a baking tray with parchment paper.

2. To prepare the vegetables, first, clean them and cut the carrots in half, if using large ones. Deseed the pepper and slice. Remove the skin of the pumpkin, parsnips, and potatoes before cutting into chunks. Cut the drained baby beetroots in half.

3. In the tray, place the vegetables in one layer and toss with a small amount of oil, salt, and pepper. Place in the oven.

4. The glaze is made by mixing the ingredients together in a bowl.

5. Baste the vegetables by coating them in a layer of glaze two to three times while cooking. Be sure to flip the vegetables halfway through the cooking process. Remove after 45 minutes, when they should be golden and crispy.

Beetroot Dip

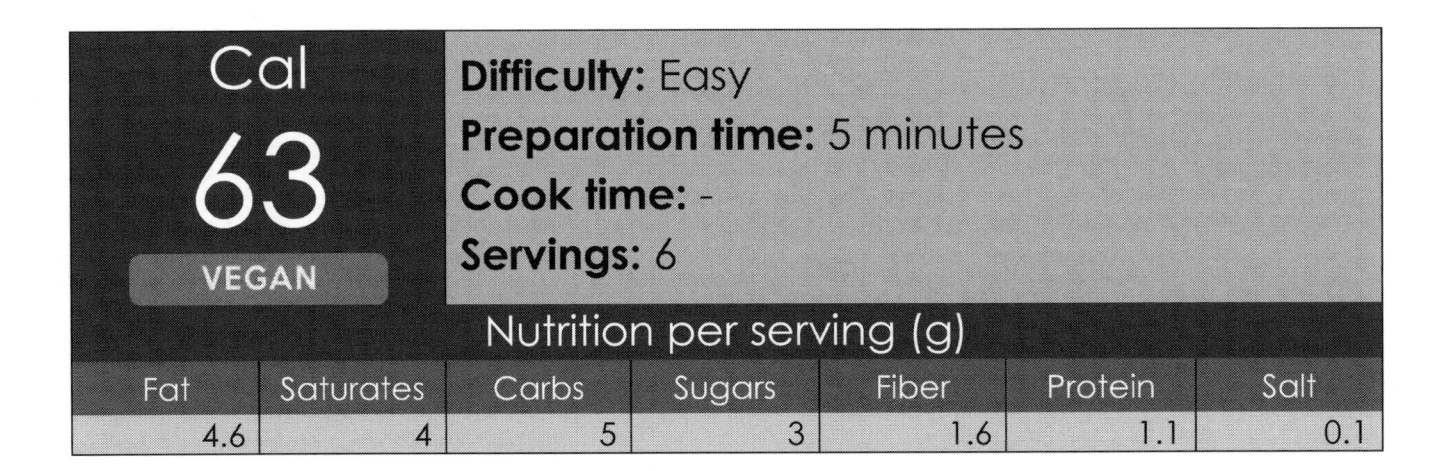

Cal **63** VEGAN	**Difficulty:** Easy **Preparation time:** 5 minutes **Cook time:** - **Servings:** 6

Nutrition per serving (g)

Fat	Saturates	Carbs	Sugars	Fiber	Protein	Salt
4.6	4	5	3	1.6	1.1	0.1

Ingredients

- 1 ¼ cups baby beetroot, canned, drained
- 1 tbsp lemon juice
- 1 cup mint leaves, unchopped
- 1 tsp cumin seeds, whole
- ½ tsp fennel seeds
- ½ tsp coriander, ground
- ½ cup coconut yogurt, or other approved yogurts

Method

1. In a blender or food processor, place the beetroot, lemon juice, coriander, cumin, and fennel. Add the yogurt to the mixture and mix until the dip is smooth and at the desired consistency. The dip will thicken when it is cooled in the fridge.

2. Serve with plain chips, fresh vegetables, or rice crackers.

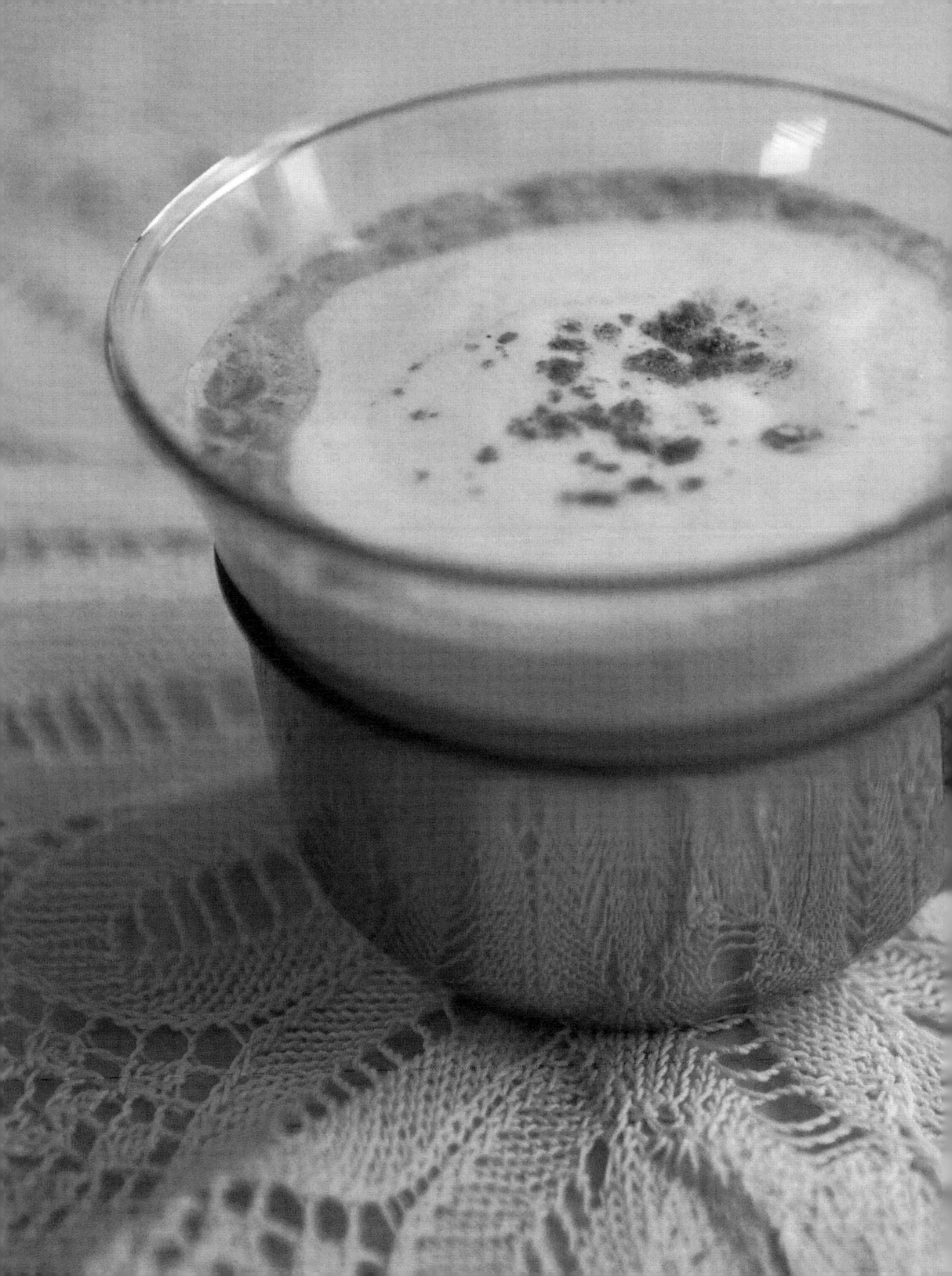

Drinks

Strawberry Basil Soda **VEGAN** 126

Raspberry Mocktail **VEGAN** 127

Electrolyte Refresher **VEGETARIAN** 128

Strawberry Lemonade **VEGAN** 129

Cranberry Lemonade **VEGAN** 130

Mock Piña Colada **VEGAN** 131

Hot Ginger and Lemon **VEGAN** 132

Spiced Hot Chocolate **VEGAN** 133

Cinnamon and Cranberry Fizz **VEGAN** 134

Golden Coffee **VEGETARIAN** 135

White Matcha Latte **VEGAN** 136

Hot Oat Milk **VEGAN** 137

Fruity Mimosa **VEGAN** 138

Strawberry Basil Soda

Cal 324 VEGAN

Difficulty: Easy
Preparation time: 5 minutes
Cook time: 10 minutes
Servings: 1

Nutrition per serving (g)

Fat	Saturates	Carbs	Sugars	Fiber	Protein	Salt
17	10	36	23	3	9	0.2

Ingredients

- ¼ cup brown sugar
- ¼ cup white sugar
- 1 cup water
- 1 cup strawberries
- ½ lemon, juiced
- 5 basil leaves
- Soda water, 1 cup per person

Method

1. Place a pot with water and sugar in it over medium heat, and bring the mixture to a simmer.

2. Add the strawberries to the pot and cook for 5 minutes, stirring occasionally to break up the strawberries. After 5 minutes, remove the mixture from the heat and allow it to cool to room temperature.

3. Add the lemon juice and the strawberry mix to a blender and blend until the syrup is smooth.

4. Serve 2 tablespoons of syrup with a cup of soda water, mixing gently. Top with ice and a small amount of basil.

Raspberry Mocktail

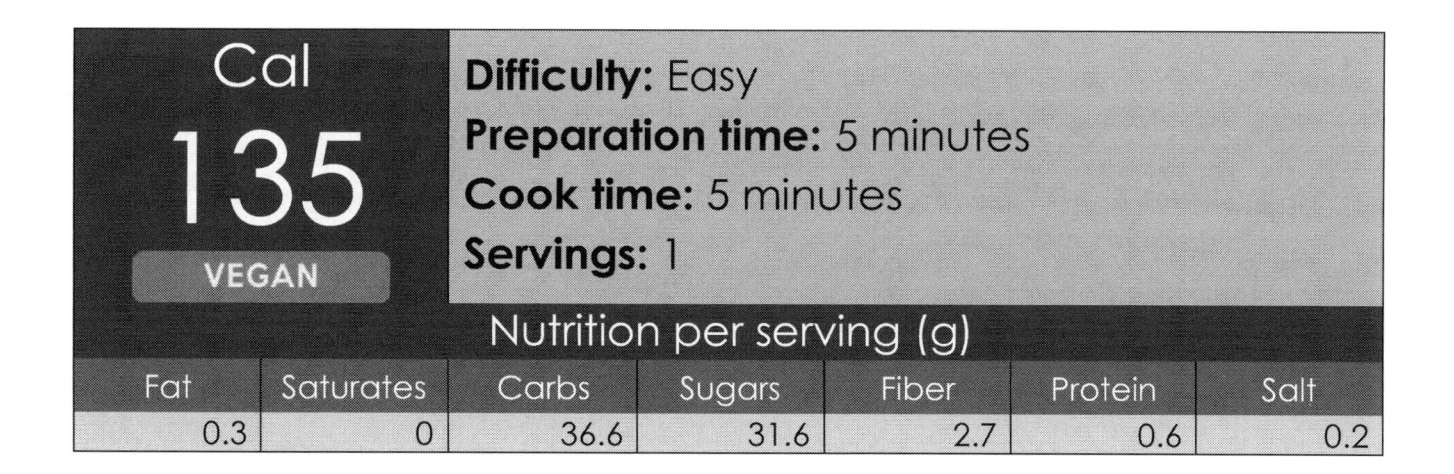

Cal 135
VEGAN

Difficulty: Easy
Preparation time: 5 minutes
Cook time: 5 minutes
Servings: 1

Nutrition per serving (g)

Fat	Saturates	Carbs	Sugars	Fiber	Protein	Salt
0.3	0	36.6	31.6	2.7	0.6	0.2

Ingredients

- 4 raspberries
- 5 mint leaves
- 2 tbsp simple syrup (instructions below: ½ cup brown sugar, ½ cup white sugar, 1 cup water)
- Ice
- ¼ cup raspberry juice
- 2 tbsp lime juice
- ½ cup soda water

Method

1. In a saucepan over medium heat, mix the water and sugar together, stirring regularly. Once the sugar is dissolved, take the mixture off the heat and allow to cool.

2. Place the raspberries, mint, and 2 tablespoons of the simple syrup in a tall glass or jam jar. Use the back of a wooden spoon to crush the ingredients. Try not to break up the mint leaves completely.

3. Add ice and lime juice to the glass and fill with soda water.

Electrolyte Refresher

Cal 67
VEGETARIAN

Difficulty: Easy
Preparation time: 5 minutes
Cook time: -
Servings: 2

Nutrition per serving (g)

Fat	Saturates	Carbs	Sugars	Fiber	Protein	Salt
0	0	18.5	17.5	0	0	0.2

Ingredients

- 1 ½ cups water
- ½ lemon, juice
- Pinch of salt
- 2 tbsp raw honey

Method

1. Mix the ingredients together in a large jar. Store in the fridge if not drinking immediately.

Strawberry Lemonade

Cal 49.5
VEGAN

Difficulty: Easy
Preparation time: 5 minutes
Cook time: 5 minutes
Servings: 2

Nutrition per serving (g)

Fat	Saturates	Carbs	Sugars	Fiber	Protein	Salt
0	0	12.5	9	1.5	0.5	0.2

Ingredients

- 1 ½ cups lemon-flavored tea
- ¾ cup frozen strawberries
- 1 tbsp lemon juice, fresh
- 1 tbsp maple syrup
- ½ cup ice cubes, optional

Method

1. Brew the tea the night before, allowing it to cool overnight.

2. Place the tea, strawberries, sugar, and lemon juice into a blender and blend. Add ice cubes until you get the desired consistency. Add extra strawberries, lemon juice, or sugar until the flavor is ideal.

3. Pour into glasses, then add ice and strawberry slices as garnish.

Cranberry Lemonade

Cal 73.5 VEGAN

Difficulty: Easy
Preparation time: 5 minutes
Cook time: 2 minutes
Servings: 4

Nutrition per serving (g)

Fat	Saturates	Carbs	Sugars	Fiber	Protein	Salt
0.5	0	18	5	7.5	2	0.2

Ingredients

- 4 cups cranberries
- 2 lemons, juiced
- 1 cup basil, chopped
- 4 cups soda water for serving (optional)
- Ice for serving

Method

1. In a blender, mix the cranberries, lemon juice, and basil until smooth.
2. Serve over ice and top with soda water if desired.

Mock Piña Colada

Cal 207
VEGAN

Difficulty: Medium
Preparation time: 5 minutes
Cook time: 30 minutes
Servings: 4

Nutrition per serving (g)

Fat	Saturates	Carbs	Sugars	Fiber	Protein	Salt
6.9	6	37.6	29.6	1.3	1.5	0

Ingredients

- 1 ½ cups water
- ⅓ cup sugar
- ½ cup coconut milk, canned
- 1 cup banana, frozen
- 1 tsp vanilla extract
- 1 cup fresh pineapple, cubed

Serving ingredients:
- Fresh pineapple, cubed
- 3 cups ice
- Mint leaves

Method

1. In a saucepan, mix the sugar into the water and bring to a boil. Once brought to a boil, remove it from the heat and place it in a container in the fridge.

2. Cube the pineapple.

3. In a blender, mix the coconut milk, sugar water, frozen banana, vanilla extract, and pineapple. Blend until the colada mix reaches a smooth consistency.

4. In a tall glass, add crushed ice and the colada mix, then top with a mint leaf.

Hot Ginger and Lemon

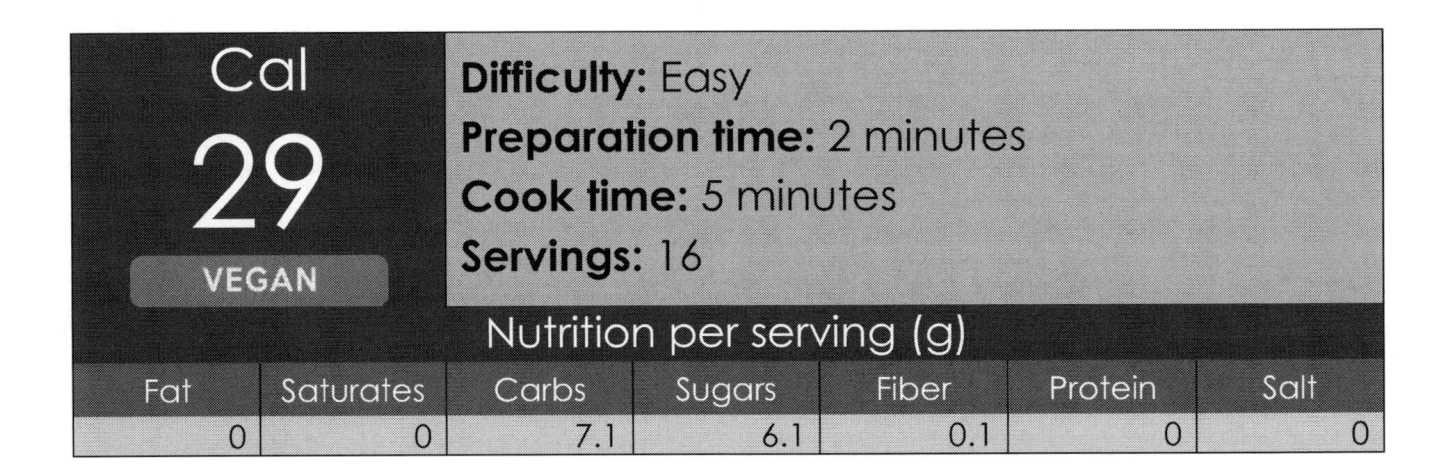

Cal 29
VEGAN

Difficulty: Easy
Preparation time: 2 minutes
Cook time: 5 minutes
Servings: 16

Nutrition per serving (g)

Fat	Saturates	Carbs	Sugars	Fiber	Protein	Salt
0	0	7.1	6.1	0.1	0	0

Ingredients

- 1 lemon
- 1 tbsp ginger, fresh
- ½ cup maple syrup

Method

1. Wash and slice the lemon, then peel and slice the ginger. Place both into a jar, layering the pieces. Pour the maple syrup over the lemon and ginger, and if desired, add more syrup to enhance the sweet flavor. Refrigerate for 12 hours overnight.

2. When serving, give the mixture a stir before putting a tablespoon into a mug and pouring hot water over it.

Spiced Hot Chocolate

Cal 349
VEGAN

Difficulty: Easy
Preparation time: 2 minutes
Cook time: 2 minutes
Servings: 2

Nutrition per serving (g)

Fat	Saturates	Carbs	Sugars	Fiber	Protein	Salt
15.5	7.5	49	28.4	4.9	3.7	0.1

Ingredients

- 2 cups lactose-free milk, or other approved milk
- ¼ cup dark chocolate
- ½ tbsp cocoa powder
- 4 tsp brown sugar
- ½ tsp vanilla extract
- 1 tsp cinnamon, ground
- 2 tsp cornstarch
- 2 tbsp water
- Pinch dried chili flakes, optional

Method

1. In a saucepan over medium heat, whisk milk, cocoa powder, sugar, vanilla, cinnamon, and a pinch of chili flakes, if desired, until the mixture is warm. Take the mixture off heat when there are no more chunks.

2. If the mixture is too thin, dissolve the corn flour in cold water and whisk into the chocolate mix. Place the mixture back over the heat to warm and thicken it. Note, it will thicken as it cools.

3. For a frothy mixture, blend for 5 seconds.

Cinnamon and Cranberry Fizz

Cal 48
VEGAN

Difficulty: Easy
Preparation time: 5 minutes
Cook time: -
Servings: 1

Nutrition per serving (g)

Fat	Saturates	Carbs	Sugars	Fiber	Protein	Salt
1	0	12	11	1	1	0.1

Ingredients

- 1 tbsp cranberry juice
- Pinch of cinnamon
- ½ cup ginger ale, ginger beer, or ginger soda water (Note: it should be sugar-free)
- Simple syrup, to taste
- Fresh cranberries and skewers, optional

Method

1. In a tall glass, pour cranberry juice, add the cinnamon, and stir.

2. Fill the glass with your choice of ginger drink and sweeten with simple syrup as desired.

3. An optional garnish is to use the skewer to thread the fresh cranberries and place them in the glass.

Golden Coffee

Cal 189
VEGETARIAN

Difficulty: Easy
Preparation time: 2 minutes
Cook time: 5 minutes
Servings: 1

Nutrition per serving (g)

Fat	Saturates	Carbs	Sugars	Fiber	Protein	Salt
8	1.5	17	10.5	5	5	0.5

Ingredients

- ½ tsp turmeric, ground
- ¼ tsp ginger, ground
- ¼ tsp cinnamon, ground
- ½ tsp black pepper, ground
- ¾ cup brewed coffee, decaffeinated
- ¼ cup coconut milk
- ½ tbsp honey

Method

1. Place the ingredients into a blender and mix well.
2. Heat through in a pot on the stove.

White Matcha Latte

Cal 178
VEGAN

Difficulty: Easy
Preparation time: 2 minutes
Cook time: 5 minutes
Servings: 1

Nutrition per serving (g)

Fat	Saturates	Carbs	Sugars	Fiber	Protein	Salt
17	8	1	1	1	2	0.2

Ingredients

- 1 ½ cups almond milk
- 1 tbsp coconut oil
- 1 bag matcha powder of choice
- ½ tsp vanilla extract

Method

1. In a saucepan over medium heat, combine the milk and coconut oil. Ensure the oil melts fully.

2. Add all the ingredients into a blender and mix until it is smooth and slightly foamy.

Hot Oat Milk

Cal 226 VEGAN	**Difficulty:** Medium **Preparation time:** 3 minutes **Cook time:** 10 minutes **Servings:** 4 ½ cups (recommended serving size is ½ cup)

Nutrition per serving (g)

Fat	Saturates	Carbs	Sugars	Fiber	Protein	Salt
5.2	0.2	33.6	2.4	5.2	5.4	0.2

Ingredients

- 1 cup rolled oats, uncooked
- 4 cups cold water
- 1 tbsp maple syrup
- 1 tsp vanilla extract
- Cheesecloth

Method

1. In a blender, mix the oats, water, maple syrup, and vanilla for 25 seconds. Do not over blend.

2. Strain the mixture through cheesecloth into a sealed jar. Do not squeeze the cloth.

3. Drink it by itself, heated, or use it in other drinks.

Fruity Mimosa

Cal 133
VEGAN

Difficulty: Easy
Preparation time: 15 minutes
Cook time: 2 minutes
Servings: 8

Nutrition per serving (g)

Fat	Saturates	Carbs	Sugars	Fiber	Protein	Salt
0.1	0	18.1	14	0.4	0.2	0

Ingredients

- ¼ cup brown sugar
- ¼ cup white sugar
- ¾ cup water
- 1 cup strawberries, fresh, chopped (Berries can be changed to other approved ones)
- 1 bottle sparkling wine

Method

1. Dissolve sugar in water for 2-3 minutes over medium heat, then cool in the fridge.

2. Blend the strawberries and sugar syrup until smooth.

3. Place 2 tablespoons of the mix into a champagne glass and top with sparkling wine.

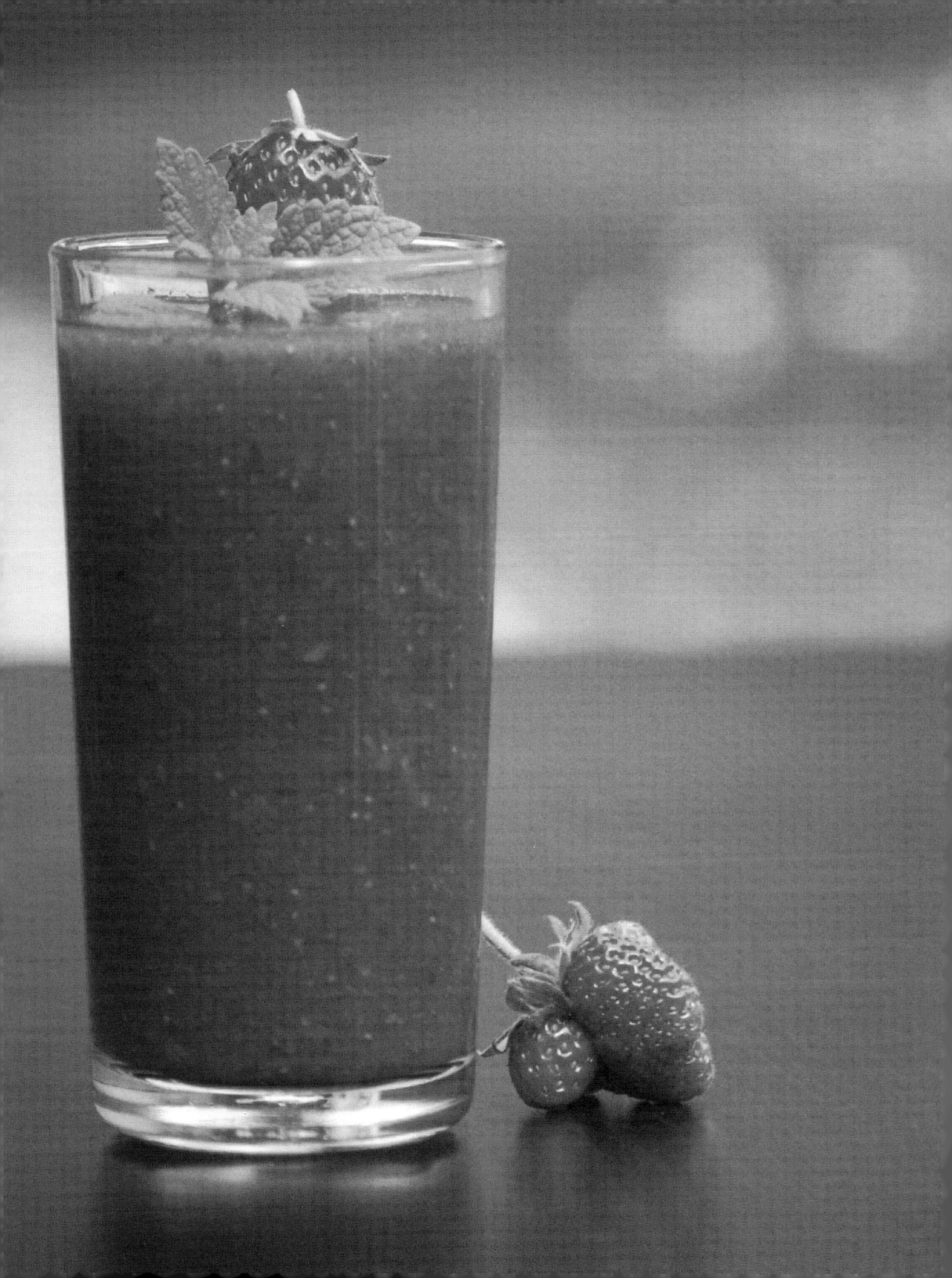

Smoothies

Basic Smoothie Base 142

Smoothie Bowl `VEGAN` 144

Kale, Ginger, and Pineapple Smoothie `VEGAN` 145

Strawberry Smoothie `VEGAN` 146

Blueberry, Lime, and Coconut Smoothie `VEGAN` 147

Pineapple, Strawberry, Raspberry Smoothie `VEGAN` .. 148

Tropical Smoothie `VEGAN` 149

Green Smoothie `VEGAN` 150

Blueberry Lime Smoothie `VEGETARIAN` 151

Blueberry, Kiwi, and Mint `VEGETARIAN` 152

Fruit Salad Smoothie `VEGETARIAN` 153

Protein Smoothie `VEGAN` 154

Cranberry Almond Bowl `VEGETARIAN` 155

Basic Smoothie Base

Difficulty: Easy
Preparation time: 2 minutes
Cook time: 3 minutes
Servings: 1

Ingredients

Base *
- 1 banana, sliced and frozen
- ¾ cup Greek yogurt
- 2 tbsp almond milk
- ¼ tsp vanilla extract
- ¼ cup ice, optional

Flavoring variations

Choconut *
- 1 tbsp peanut butter
- 1 tbsp cocoa powder
- Pinch of salt

Berry *
- ½ cup strawberries, can be replaced with any other approved berry or a mixture
- 5 mint leaves
- Pinch of salt

Tropical *
- 1 cup papaya, peeled and diced
- 1 tbsp lime juice
- Pinch of salt

Method

1. In a blender, add the base ingredients and one of the flavor combinations.
2. If ice is added, drink immediately or cover and put in the fridge.

Cal 334 — Base *

Nutrition per serving (g)

Fat	Saturates	Carbs	Sugars	Fiber	Protein	Salt
17	10	36	23	3	9	0.5

Cal 430 — Base + Choconut *

Nutrition per serving (g)

Fat	Saturates	Carbs	Sugars	Fiber	Protein	Salt
26	13	42	24	6	14	0.3

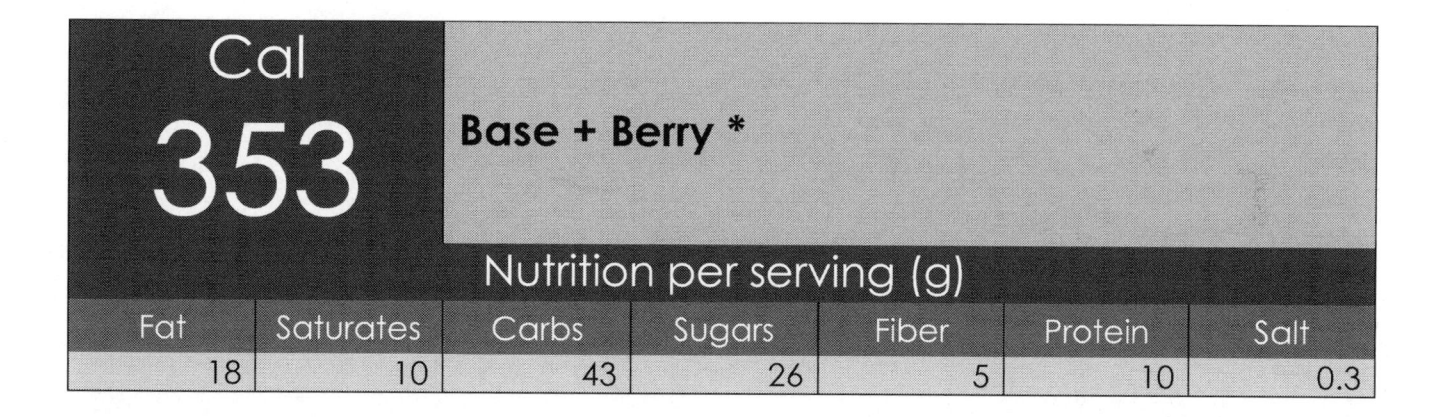

Cal 353 — Base + Berry *

Nutrition per serving (g)

Fat	Saturates	Carbs	Sugars	Fiber	Protein	Salt
18	10	43	26	5	10	0.3

Cal 383 — Base + Tropical *

Nutrition per serving (g)

Fat	Saturates	Carbs	Sugars	Fiber	Protein	Salt
18	11	51	31	6	10	0.2

Smoothie Bowl

Cal 324 — VEGAN

Difficulty: Easy
Preparation time: 5 minutes
Cook time: 5 minutes
Servings: 2

Nutrition per serving (g)

Fat	Saturates	Carbs	Sugars	Fiber	Protein	Salt
17	10	36	23	3	9	0.5

Ingredients

- 1 cup coconut yogurt
- ½ cup coconut milk, canned or fresh
- 4 bananas, cut into slices and frozen
- 2 cups frozen mixed berries
- 2 tsp lemon juice
- ½ cup mixed nuts, chopped
- 2 mint leaves, torn

Method

1. In a blender, mix yogurt, milk, bananas, frozen berries, and lemon juice.
2. Pour the mix into bowls and top with nuts and mint.

Kale, Ginger, and Pineapple Smoothie

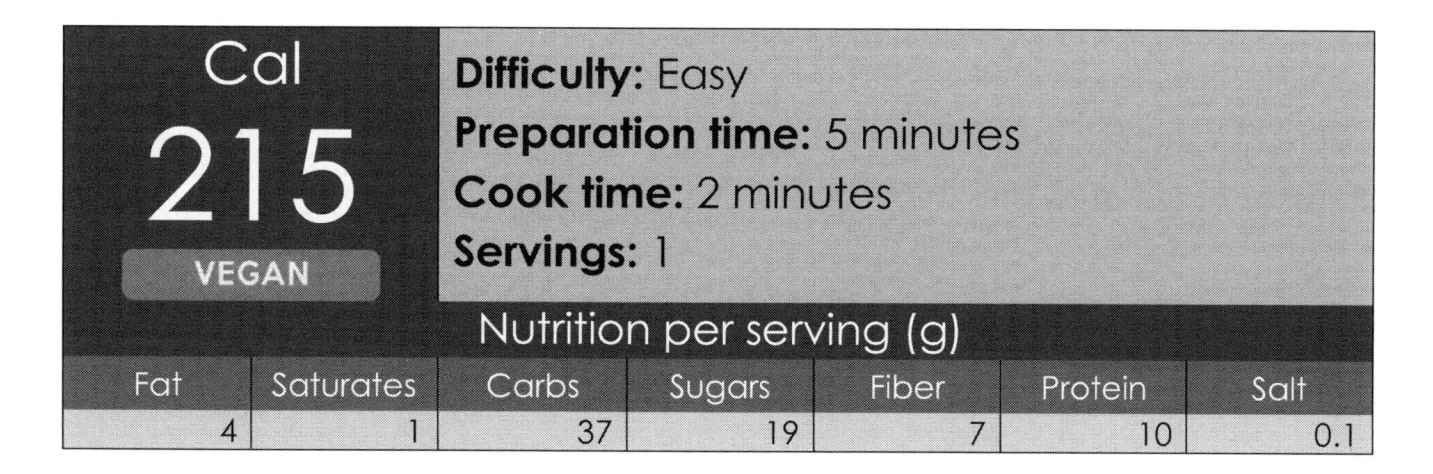

Cal 215
VEGAN

Difficulty: Easy
Preparation time: 5 minutes
Cook time: 2 minutes
Servings: 1

Nutrition per serving (g)

Fat	Saturates	Carbs	Sugars	Fiber	Protein	Salt
4	1	37	19	7	10	0.1

Ingredients

- 1 cup FODMAP-approved milk (lactose-free or coconut)
- ½ peeled orange
- ¾ cup pineapple, fresh or frozen
- 1 cup raw kale
- Pinch of ground ginger
- 1 cup ice

Method

Place ingredients in a blender and blend until smooth.

Strawberry Smoothie

Cal 308
VEGAN

Difficulty: Easy
Preparation time: 2 minutes
Cook time: 3 minutes
Servings: 1

Nutrition per serving (g)

Fat	Saturates	Carbs	Sugars	Fiber	Protein	Salt
10.3	1.4	1.4	30.9	5.9	5.4	0.2

Ingredients

- ½ cup FODMAP-approved milk (almond milk is recommended)
- ⅔ cup strawberries, fresh or frozen
- ¼ cup lactose-free yogurt or vegan yogurt
- 1 ½ tsp protein powder
- 1 tsp chia seeds
- ½ tbsp maple syrup
- 1 tsp lemon juice
- ¼ tsp vanilla extract
- 6 ice cubes (only when using fresh strawberries)

Method

1 Cut the strawberries into halves or quarters. If using frozen strawberries, it is recommended to cut them the day before.

2 Put ingredients into a blender and blend until smooth. If the mixture gets too thick, add a small amount of hot water and continue blending.

3 It is best drunk immediately.

Blueberry, Lime, and Coconut Smoothie

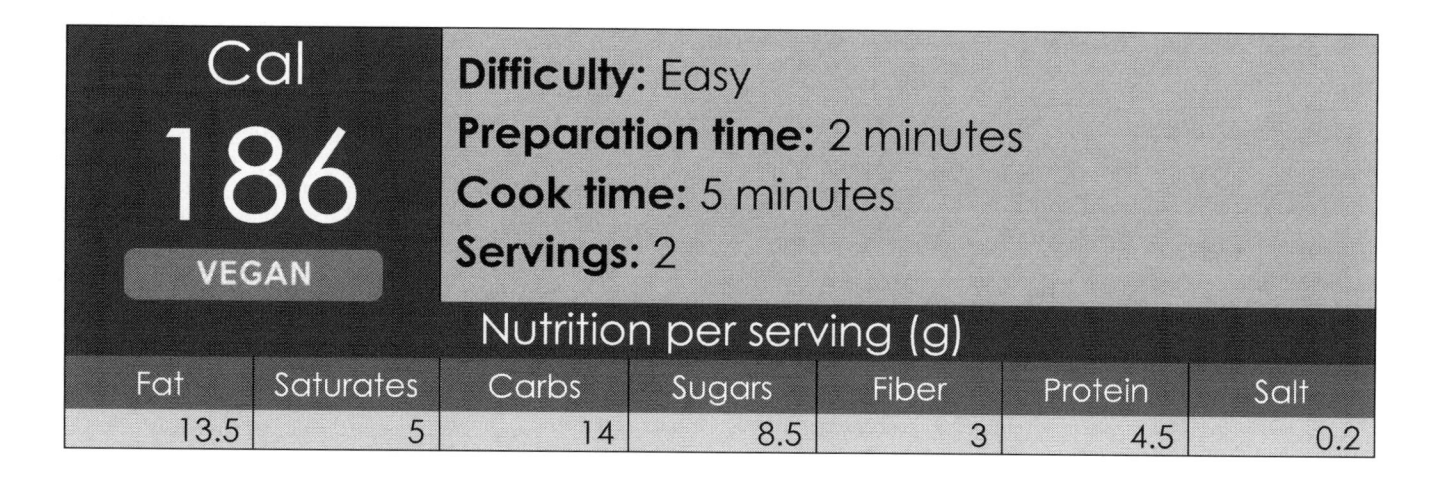

Cal 186
VEGAN

Difficulty: Easy
Preparation time: 2 minutes
Cook time: 5 minutes
Servings: 2

Nutrition per serving (g)

Fat	Saturates	Carbs	Sugars	Fiber	Protein	Salt
13.5	5	14	8.5	3	4.5	0.2

Ingredients

- ½ cup blueberries, fresh or frozen
- 2 tbsp coconut flakes
- 2 tbsp lime juice
- ⅔ cup FODMAP-approved yogurt or vegan yogurt
- 1 tsp chia seeds
- 2 tbsp water
- Ice, when using fresh blueberries (Approximately 6 cubes, depending on the desired texture)

Method

Blend all ingredients together until frothy.

Pineapple, Strawberry, Raspberry Smoothie

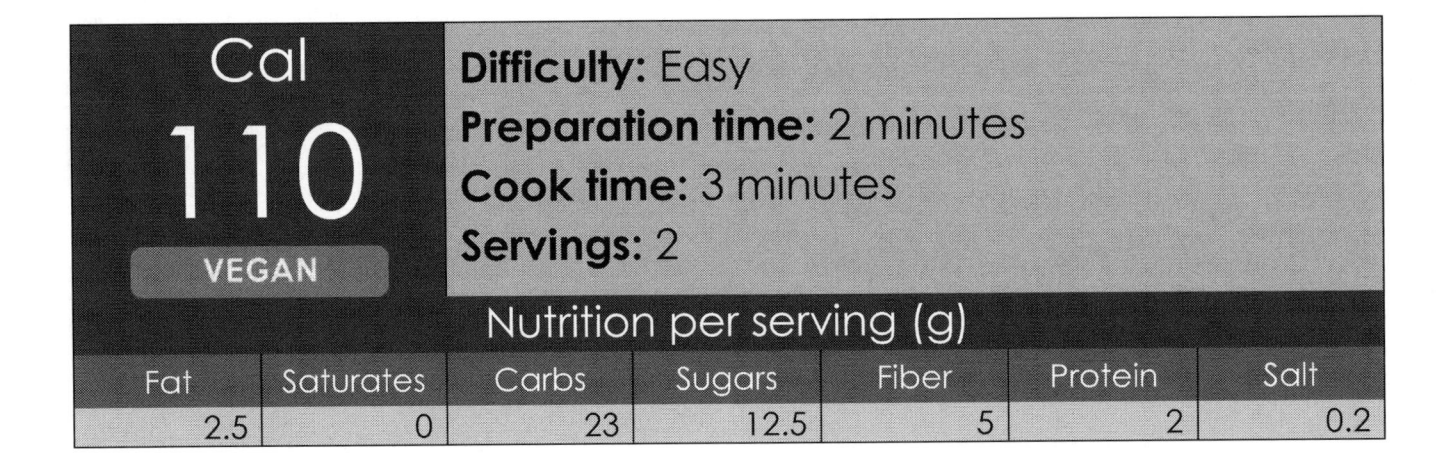

Cal 110
VEGAN

Difficulty: Easy
Preparation time: 2 minutes
Cook time: 3 minutes
Servings: 2

Nutrition per serving (g)

Fat	Saturates	Carbs	Sugars	Fiber	Protein	Salt
2.5	0	23	12.5	5	2	0.2

Ingredients

- 1 banana, frozen and sliced
- ½ cup strawberries, fresh or frozen
- ¼ cup pineapple, fresh
- ½ cup raspberries, frozen
- 1 cup almond milk, can substitute other approved milk

Method

Place ingredients in a blender and blend. Add more milk to create a thinner consistency.

Tropical Smoothie

Cal 434
VEGAN

Difficulty: Easy
Preparation time: 2 minutes
Cook time: 3 minutes
Servings: 1

Nutrition per serving (g)

Fat	Saturates	Carbs	Sugars	Fiber	Protein	Salt
28	22	44	20	7	7	0.2

Ingredients

- ¾ cup frozen pineapple
- 1 cup baby spinach
- ½ tbsp lime juice
- ¾ cup ginger, ground
- ½ cup oat milk
- ½ cup coconut milk
- 1 tbsp flaxseed
- Pinch of salt

Method

Mix the ingredients in a blender. Once the mixture has a smooth consistency, enjoy!

Green Smoothie

Cal 121
VEGAN

Difficulty: Easy
Preparation time: 3 minutes
Cook time: 3 minutes
Servings: 1

Nutrition per serving (g)

Fat	Saturates	Carbs	Sugars	Fiber	Protein	Salt
3	0	22	12	6	4	0.2

Ingredients

- ½ cup spinach
- ½ cup kale
- 1 orange, peeled
- 1 tbsp flaxseed
- 1 tbsp ginger, juice or ground
- 1 cup water (add more or less depending on the desired consistency)

Method

Combine the ingredients in a blender, then blend to the desired consistency.

Blueberry Lime Smoothie

Cal **319** VEGETARIAN	**Difficulty:** Easy **Preparation time:** 2 minutes **Cook time:** 3 minutes **Servings:** 1

Nutrition per serving (g)

Fat	Saturates	Carbs	Sugars	Fiber	Protein	Salt
23	7	26	15	6	7	0

Ingredients

- ½ cup blueberries, fresh or frozen
- 2 tbsp coconut flakes
- 2 tbsp lime juice, fresh
- ½ cup Greek or lactose-free yogurt
- 1 tsp chia seeds
- 2 tbsp water
- Ice (only if using fresh blueberries and if you want a thicker consistency)

Method

Place ingredients in a blender and mix until it starts to look frothy.

Blueberry, Kiwi, and Mint

Cal 226
VEGETARIAN

Difficulty: Easy
Preparation time: 3 minutes
Cook time: 3 minutes
Servings: 1

Nutrition per serving (g)

Fat	Saturates	Carbs	Sugars	Fiber	Protein	Salt
12	7	27	19	4	6	0

Ingredients

- ½ cup blueberries, frozen
- 1 kiwi, small, peeled
- ⅓ cup Greek yogurt
- ⅓ cup water
- 6 mint leaves, fresh

Method

Mix the ingredients in a blender until creamy.

Fruit Salad Smoothie

Cal 129.5
VEGETARIAN

Difficulty: Easy
Preparation time: 3 minutes
Cook time: 5 minutes
Servings: 2

Nutrition per serving (g)

Fat	Saturates	Carbs	Sugars	Fiber	Protein	Salt
8	3	15.5	11	2.5	2	0.2

Ingredients

- 1 cup canned fruit salad, frozen
- 2 tbsp lactose-free yogurt
- 2 tbsp coconut milk
- 2 tsp coconut, shredded
- 2 tsp walnuts, chopped finely
- 1 tsp lemon zest, optional
- ½ cup water to thin out the mixture

Method

1. Blend together fruit, yogurt, milk, water, and lemon zest until smooth.
2. Add water to thin out the consistency, if desired.
3. Top with shredded coconut and walnuts.

Protein Smoothie

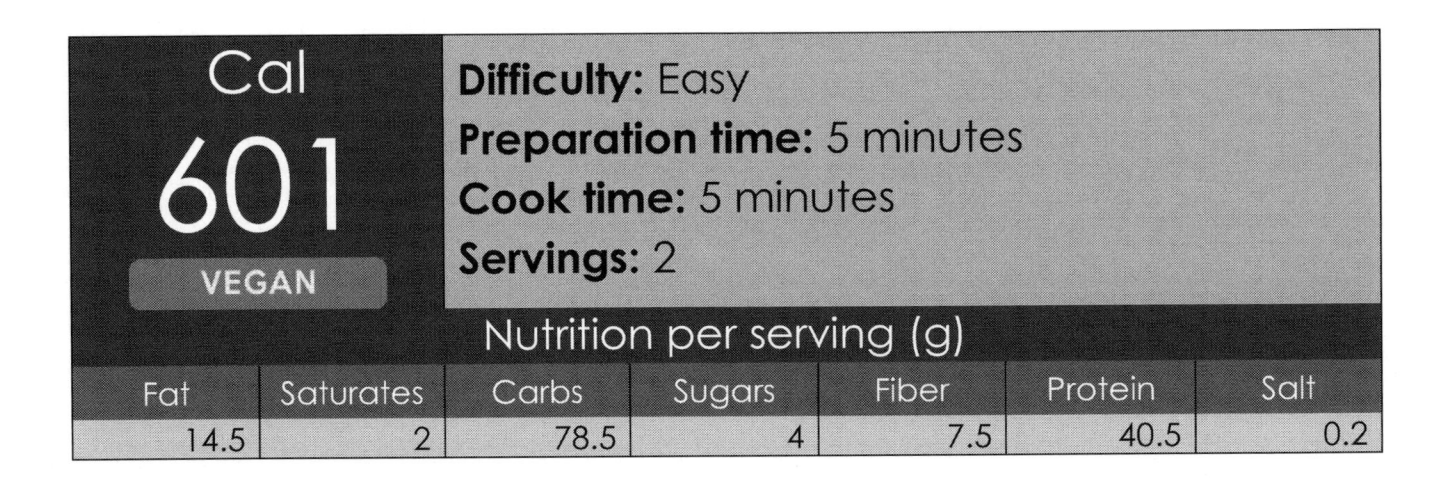

Cal 601
VEGAN

Difficulty: Easy
Preparation time: 5 minutes
Cook time: 5 minutes
Servings: 2

Nutrition per serving (g)

Fat	Saturates	Carbs	Sugars	Fiber	Protein	Salt
14.5	2	78.5	4	7.5	40.5	0.2

Ingredients

- ½ banana
- 1 cup vanilla protein powder
- 1 cup almond milk
- 1 ½ tbsp drinking chocolate
- 1 ½ cups ice cubes

Method

1. Add all the ingredients, except the ice, into a blender and mix together.
2. Add the ice slowly until the mixture is creamy.

Cranberry Almond Bowl

Cal 545 — VEGETARIAN

Difficulty: Easy
Preparation time: 2 minutes
Cook time: 2 minutes
Servings: 1

Nutrition per serving (g)

Fat	Saturates	Carbs	Sugars	Fiber	Protein	Salt
30	9	65	24	22	13	0

Ingredients

- 1 cup cranberries, frozen
- 1 tbsp almond butter
- ½ cup Greek yogurt
- 2 tbsp lactose-free milk
- ½ small banana, frozen
- 1 tbsp chia seeds
- ½ cup ice cubes
- Optional toppings, chopped nuts

Method

1. Blend together cranberries, butter, Greek yogurt, milk, banana, and chia seeds.

2. Add ice until the desired consistency is achieved.

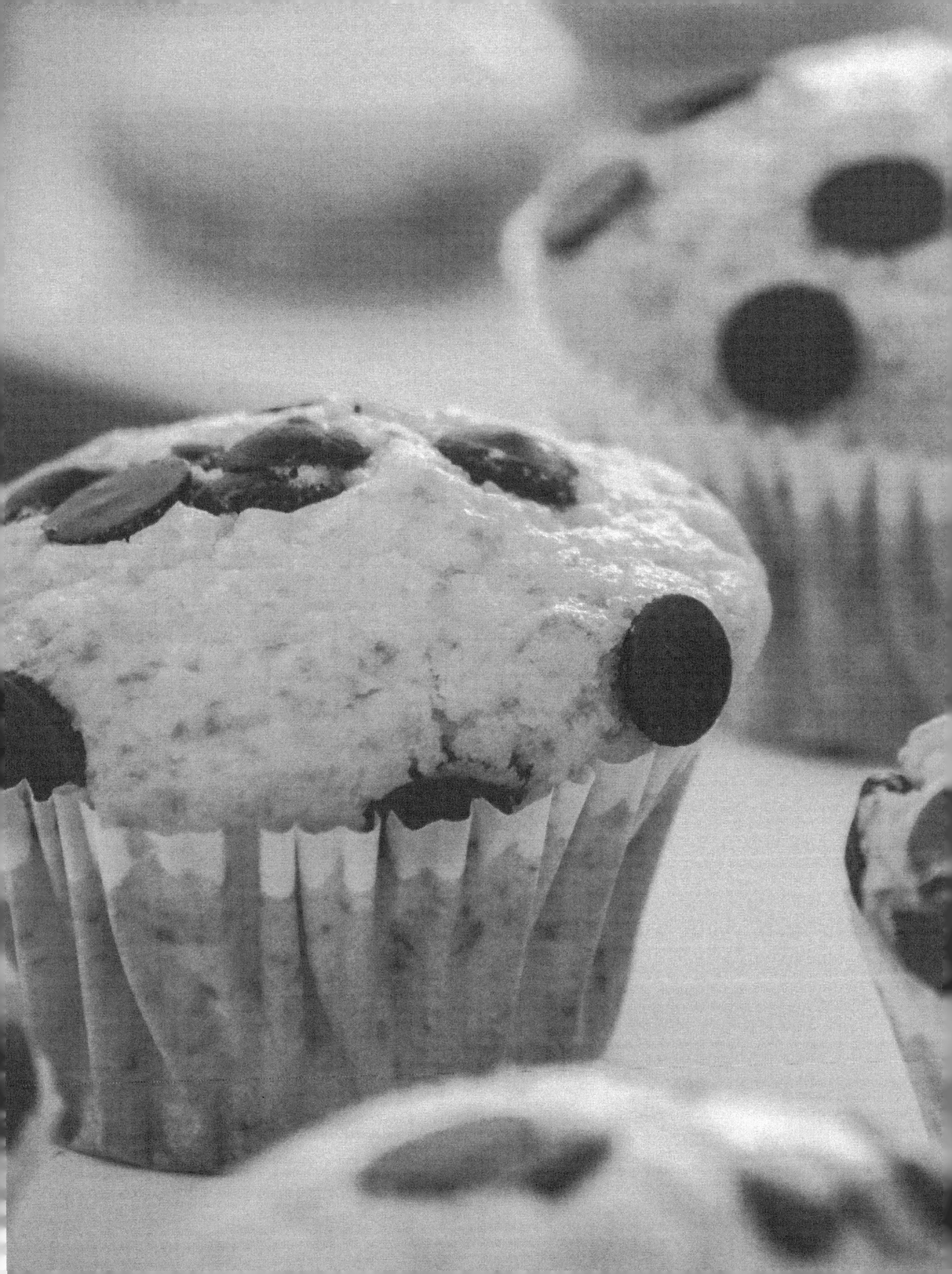

Snacks

Sweet and Savory Popcorn `VEGAN` 158

Quinoa Muffins `VEGETARIAN` 159

Lemon Coconut Cupcakes `VEGETARIAN` 160

Chocolate Peanut Butter Energy Bites `VEGAN` 161

Blueberry Muffins `VEGAN` 162

Summer Popsicle `VEGAN` 163

Pineapple, Yogurt on Rice Cakes `VEGETARIAN` 164

Salted Caramel Pumpkin Seeds `VEGETARIAN` 165

Orange Biscuits `VEGETARIAN` 166

Coconut Bites `VEGETARIAN` 167

Carrot Parsnip Chips `VEGAN` 168

Baked Oat Cup `VEGETARIAN` 169

Energy Bars `VEGETARIAN` 170

Sweet and Savory Popcorn

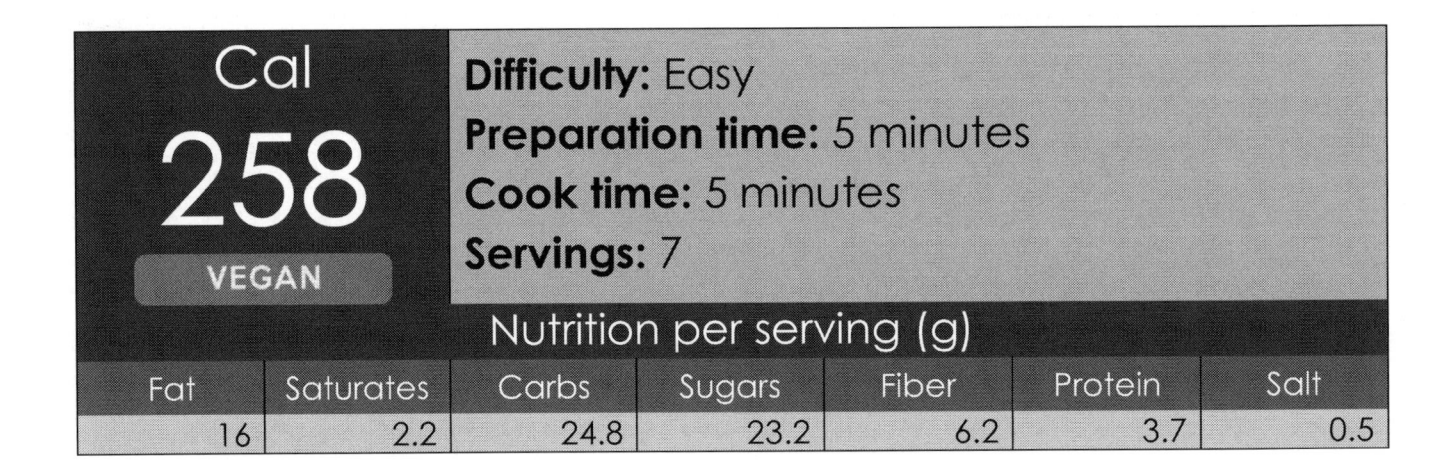

Cal 258 VEGAN

Difficulty: Easy
Preparation time: 5 minutes
Cook time: 5 minutes
Servings: 7

Nutrition per serving (g)

Fat	Saturates	Carbs	Sugars	Fiber	Protein	Salt
16	2.2	24.8	23.2	6.2	3.7	0.5

Ingredients

- ½ cup vegetable oil
- 1 cup popcorn kernels
- ⅓ cup brown sugar
- ⅓ cup white sugar
- 2 tsp salt, or to taste

Method

1. Blend together cranberries, butter, Greek yogurt, milk, banana, and chia seeds.

2. Add ice until the desired consistency is achieved.

Quinoa Muffins

Cal 175 — VEGETARIAN

Difficulty: Easy
Preparation time: 10 minutes
Cook time: 20 minutes
Servings: 24 muffins (1 per serving)

Nutrition per serving (g)

Fat	Saturates	Carbs	Sugars	Fiber	Protein	Salt
10.5	4	6	4	1.5	14	0.5

Ingredients

- 1 ½ cups quinoa flour
- 1 cup quinoa flakes
- ⅓ cup walnuts, chopped
- 1 tbsp cinnamon
- 4 tsp baking powder
- 2 tsp baking soda
- Pinch of salt
- 4 eggs
- 4 bananas, mashed
- ½ cup almond milk
- ¼ cup maple syrup

Method

1. Preheat the oven to 375°F.

2. Mix the dry ingredients in one bowl. In a separate bowl, combine the wet ingredients. Combine the ingredients until mixed fully.

3. Spoon into greased muffin pans and bake for 20 minutes. Check if the center is dry by poking the center of a muffin with a skewer. If it comes out clean, they are ready.

Lemon Coconut Cupcakes

Cal 366 VEGETARIAN

Difficulty: Medium
Preparation time: 25 minutes
Cook time: 25 minutes
Servings: 12

Nutrition per serving (g)

Fat	Saturates	Carbs	Sugars	Fiber	Protein	Salt
17.5	4.4	49.4	34.3	0.4	2.7	0.3

Ingredients

Cupcakes
- 1 ½ cups gluten-free, all-purpose flour
- ½ tsp xanthan gum
- 2 tsp of baking powder
- Pinch of salt
- 1 tbsp lemon zest
- ½ cup butter, room temperature
- ½ cup white sugar
- ½ cup brown sugar
- 2 eggs
- 1 tsp vanilla extract
- 2 ½ tbsp lemon juice
- ½ cup coconut yogurt

Lemon butter icing
- ¾ cup butter
- 1 ½ cups powdered sugar
- 1 ½ tbsp lemon juice

Method

1. Preheat the oven to 350°F and grease a 12-muffin tin.

2. For the cupcakes, mix together the dry ingredients and put to the side.

3. In a large bowl, mix the butter and sugar until combined, then whisk together the eggs and vanilla until smooth before adding the lemon juice and blending. Add the dry ingredients and yogurt, alternating between them, beginning and ending with the dry ingredients. Mix well.

4. Spoon into muffin cups, filling ⅔ of the way. Place into the center of the oven and bake for 25 minutes. The tops should be golden. When a skewer or toothpick is inserted into them, it should come out clean. Leave to cool.

5. The icing is optional. To make the icing, mix room temperature butter and powdered sugar together with lemon juice until smooth. Then, use a knife to cover the top of the cupcakes after they have cooled.

Chocolate Peanut Butter Energy Bites

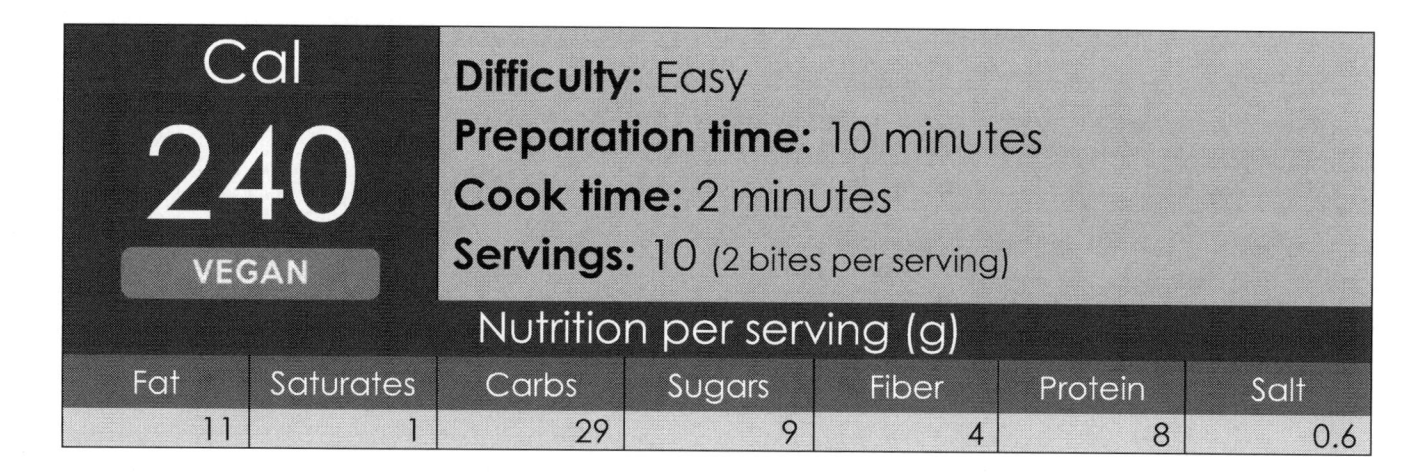

Cal 240
VEGAN

Difficulty: Easy
Preparation time: 10 minutes
Cook time: 2 minutes
Servings: 10 (2 bites per serving)

Nutrition per serving (g)

Fat	Saturates	Carbs	Sugars	Fiber	Protein	Salt
11	1	29	9	4	8	0.6

Ingredients

- ½ cup smooth peanut butter
- 1 cup oats
- ⅓ cup maple syrup
- ¼ cup peanuts, roasted, chopped
- ¼ cup dark chocolate, 55%, finely chopped
- Pinch of salt

Method

1. In a bowl, mix the ingredients.

2. Once mixed, roll the mixture into balls (approximately 1 tablespoon in size, add more if there is mixture left once 10 balls have been rolled). They will need to be compressed as they are rolled. Store in an airtight container.

Blueberry Muffins

Cal 533
VEGAN

Difficulty: Easy
Preparation time: 15 minutes
Cook time: 30 minutes
Servings: 24 (1 muffin per serving)

Nutrition per serving (g)

Fat	Saturates	Carbs	Sugars	Fiber	Protein	Salt
34	20	54.5	27.6	3	4	0.3

Ingredients

Topping
- ½ cup oats
- 2 tbsp pecans, chopped
- 2 tbsp flour (fodmap approved)
- 2 tbsp unsalted butter, melted
- 2 tbsp brown sugar

Muffins
- 2 cups flour (fodmap approved)
- 1 cup oat flour
- 1 ½ cups brown sugar
- 1 ½ cups white sugar
- Pinch of salt
- 1 cup lactose-free milk
- ¼ cup maple syrup
- 4 cups unsalted butter, melted
- 2 cups blueberries, fresh

Method

1. Preheat the oven to 375ºF and line muffin tins with paper liners. Spray with non-stick spray.

2. In a blender, add the topping ingredients, pulse 5 times, and move to a bowl in the fridge.

3. Add the dry muffin ingredients (gluten-free flour, oat flour, sugars, salt) in a medium bowl and mix. Whisk the wet ingredients (milk, syrup, butter) together in a separate bowl. Slowly mix the dry ingredients into the wet ones. Fold the blueberries into the mixture.

4. In the muffin tins, scoop ¼ cup of batter, then crumble the topping over the mixture. Bake for 25-30 minutes. Cool for 10 minutes before removing from tin.

Summer Popsicle

Cal **156** VEGAN	**Difficulty:** Easy **Preparation time:** 15 minutes **Cook time:** 2 minutes **Servings:** 4 (5 ½ tbsp per popsicle)

Nutrition per serving (g)

Fat	Saturates	Carbs	Sugars	Fiber	Protein	Salt
0.5	0.1	38.9	19.2	9.7	2.7	0.1

Ingredients

- 4 carrots, large
- 3 oranges, large
- 1 lime, juiced
- 1 tsp orange zest
- 2 tbsp powdered sugar

Method

1. Grate the carrots.

2. In a clean cloth, wrap the carrots and squeeze the juice into a bowl.

3. Zest an orange. Juice the oranges and lime into the bowl of carrot juice and mix the zest in. Add the powdered sugar. If the mixture tastes too sour, add more powdered sugar, then pour into popsicle molds.

4. Place in the freezer overnight. If using wooden sticks, place them in after 2 hours in the freezer.

Pineapple, Yogurt on Rice Cakes

Cal 169
VEGETARIAN

Difficulty: Easy
Preparation time: 5 minutes
Cook time: 12 minutes
Servings: 1 (2 rice cakes)

Nutrition per serving (g)

Fat	Saturates	Carbs	Sugars	Fiber	Protein	Salt
1.5	0.4	35.6	10	1.5	3.8	0

Ingredients

- 2 rice cakes
- ⅓ cup fresh pineapple, sliced
- 2 tbsp Greek yogurt
- ¼ tsp chia seeds, optional
- 1 tsp oil, used to prevent the pineapple from burning

Method

1. Spray the pineapple slices with oil, then place them on a tray in the oven and bake for 5 minutes on each side. Cut into chunky pieces.

2. Spread the yogurt over the rice cake and top with pineapple and chia seeds.

Salted Caramel Pumpkin Seeds

Cal 124
VEGETARIAN

Difficulty: Easy
Preparation time: 5 minutes
Cook time: 25 minutes
Servings: 16 (2 tbsp per serving)

Nutrition per serving (g)

Fat	Saturates	Carbs	Sugars	Fiber	Protein	Salt
9.8	1.7	5.7	4	1.1	5.4	0.1

Ingredients

Roasted seeds
- 2 cups pumpkin seeds
- 2 ½ tbsp sugar
- ¼ tsp cinnamon, ground
- ½ tsp ginger, ground
- Pinch of nutmeg
- 2 tsp water

Salted caramel sauce
- 1 ½ tbsp butter
- 1 tbsp white sugar
- 1 ½ tbsp brown sugar
- ½ tsp rock salt

Method

1. Preheat the oven to 300ºF.

2. Mix the pumpkin seeds, spices, and sugar with water. The seeds should be damp to allow the spices and sugar to stick.

3. Line a tray with parchment paper and grease it. Spread the seeds evenly over the tray, then bake in the oven for 25 minutes. The seeds should be golden and crunchy. Remember to mix the seeds up halfway through cooking.

4. When the seeds finish baking, place a saucepan over medium heat and melt the butter. Mix the sugar and salt into the butter, then cook for 2 minutes until the mixture is a deep golden color. Lower the heat. Mix the seeds into the caramel, transfer back to the tray, and let cool.

Orange Biscuits

Cal 154
VEGETARIAN

Difficulty: Easy
Preparation time: 25 minutes
Cook time: 25 minutes
Servings: 24 (1-2 per serving)

Nutrition per serving (g)

Fat	Saturates	Carbs	Sugars	Fiber	Protein	Salt
4.1	0.6	27.8	14.6	1.7	1.3	0.1

Ingredients

Biscuits
- ½ tsp of baking soda
- Pinch of salt
- 2 cups flour, gluten-free or oat
- 1 tsp orange zest
- ½ cup butter
- ½ cup brown sugar
- ½ cup white sugar
- 1 egg, large
- 2 tbsp orange juice, fresh
- 1 tsp vanilla extract

Glaze
- 1 cup powdered sugar
- 1 ½ tsp orange zest
- 1 ½ tbsp orange juice, fresh

Method

1. Preheat the oven to 350°F.

2. Use a grater to zest the orange. Do not grate the white layer.

3. Whisk the salt, baking soda, zest, and flour together in a large bowl.

4. In a different bowl, beat the butter and sugar together using an electric hand beater until the mixture is fluffy and not grainy. Add 2 tablespoons of orange juice, the egg, and the vanilla to the mixture.

5. Combine the dry and wet ingredients and mix until the dough is sticky. Form balls using about 2 tablespoons of dough. Place the balls on trays that are covered in parchment paper, then flatten the dough slightly before baking for 15-20 minutes. Rotate the trays halfway through. When the edges are golden brown, remove the trays and let them cool down on cooling racks.

6. For the icing, mix the powdered sugar, orange juice, and zest together. The icing should be sticky and not runny. Use a teaspoon to ice the biscuits once they are cool.

Coconut Bites

Cal 139 VEGETARIAN

Difficulty: Easy
Preparation time: 15 minutes
Cook time: 2 minutes
Servings: 14 (4 bites per serving)

Nutrition per serving (g)

Fat	Saturates	Carbs	Sugars	Fiber	Protein	Salt
8.2	2.5	14.9	8	0.8	1.8	0.1

Ingredients

- 2 cups cornflakes, gluten-free
- ½ cup brown sugar
- ¼ cup oats
- 6 tbsp dried coconut, shredded
- 4 tbsp pumpkin seeds
- 6 tbsp butter

Method

1. Crush the cornflakes and soften the butter. Place all the ingredients, except the coconut, into a food processor and pulse until large crumbs form.

2. Press and roll the mixture into balls, approximately 1 tbsp per ball (add more if there is leftover dough), then roll in the coconut.

3. Store in the fridge.

Carrot Parsnip Chips

Cal 386 VEGAN

Difficulty: Easy
Preparation time: 5 minutes
Cook time: 35 minutes
Servings: 3

Nutrition per serving (g)

Fat	Saturates	Carbs	Sugars	Fiber	Protein	Salt
10	1	73	24	20	6	0.3

Ingredients

- 1 large parsnip, peeled and ends cut off
- 1 large carrot, peeled and ends cut off
- 2 tsp olive oil
- Pinch of salt
- 1 tsp thyme leaves

Method

1. Preheat the oven to 325°F.
2. Oil a baking tray lightly.
3. Peel the carrot and parsnip into long thin pieces and place onto the tray. Drizzle with oil and season.
4. Cook for 35 minutes, turning the vegetables 2 times during cooking.

Baked Oat Cup

Cal 206 VEGETARIAN

Difficulty: Easy
Preparation time: 5 minutes
Cook time: 25 minutes
Servings: 12 (1 per serving)

Nutrition per serving (g)

Fat	Saturates	Carbs	Sugars	Fiber	Protein	Salt
6	1.4	31.5	9	3.6	6.5	0.3

Ingredients

- 2 eggs
- 2 tbsp vegetable oil
- ½ cup water
- 1 cup lactose-free milk
- 2 tsp vanilla extract
- ⅓ cup brown sugar
- 2 ½ cups oats
- 2 tsp of baking powder
- 1 tsp cinnamon, ground
- Toppings: sliced strawberries and almonds, cranberries and walnuts, dark chocolate chips or shavings

Method

1. Preheat the oven to 350°F.
2. Line a muffin tin with paper liners.
3. Whisk the eggs, milk, and oil together in a bowl. Stir in the vanilla, sugar, oats, baking powder, and cinnamon. Leave the batter to thicken for a few minutes before stirring again.
4. Pour the batter evenly into muffin tin cups. Do not fill completely.
5. Add toppings then bake for 25 minutes.

Energy Bars

Cal 121
VEGETARIAN

Difficulty: Easy
Preparation time: 10 minutes
Cook time: -
Servings: 14 (1 slice per serving)

Nutrition per serving (g)

Fat	Saturates	Carbs	Sugars	Fiber	Protein	Salt
6.4	1	14.4	8.8	1.2	3	0

Ingredients

- ⅓ cup sunflower seed butter or peanut butter
- 6 tbsp maple syrup
- 1 ½ cups puffed rice
- ½ cup pumpkin seeds, roughly chopped
- 4 tbsp dried cranberries, chopped roughly
- ½ tsp ginger, ground
- ½ tsp cinnamon, ground
- 1 tbsp dark chocolate, chopped roughly

Method

1. Line a square baking pan with parchment paper.

2. Melt the butter and the syrup over medium heat. Once melted, remove from the heat and stir in the pumpkin seeds, puffed rice, dried cranberries, ginger, and cinnamon. Coat the ingredients evenly.

3. Spread the mixture across the pan evenly, then place another piece of parchment paper over the mixture and apply pressure evenly to compress.

4. Melt the dark chocolate, then drizzle over the mixture. Refrigerate for 2 hours before cutting.

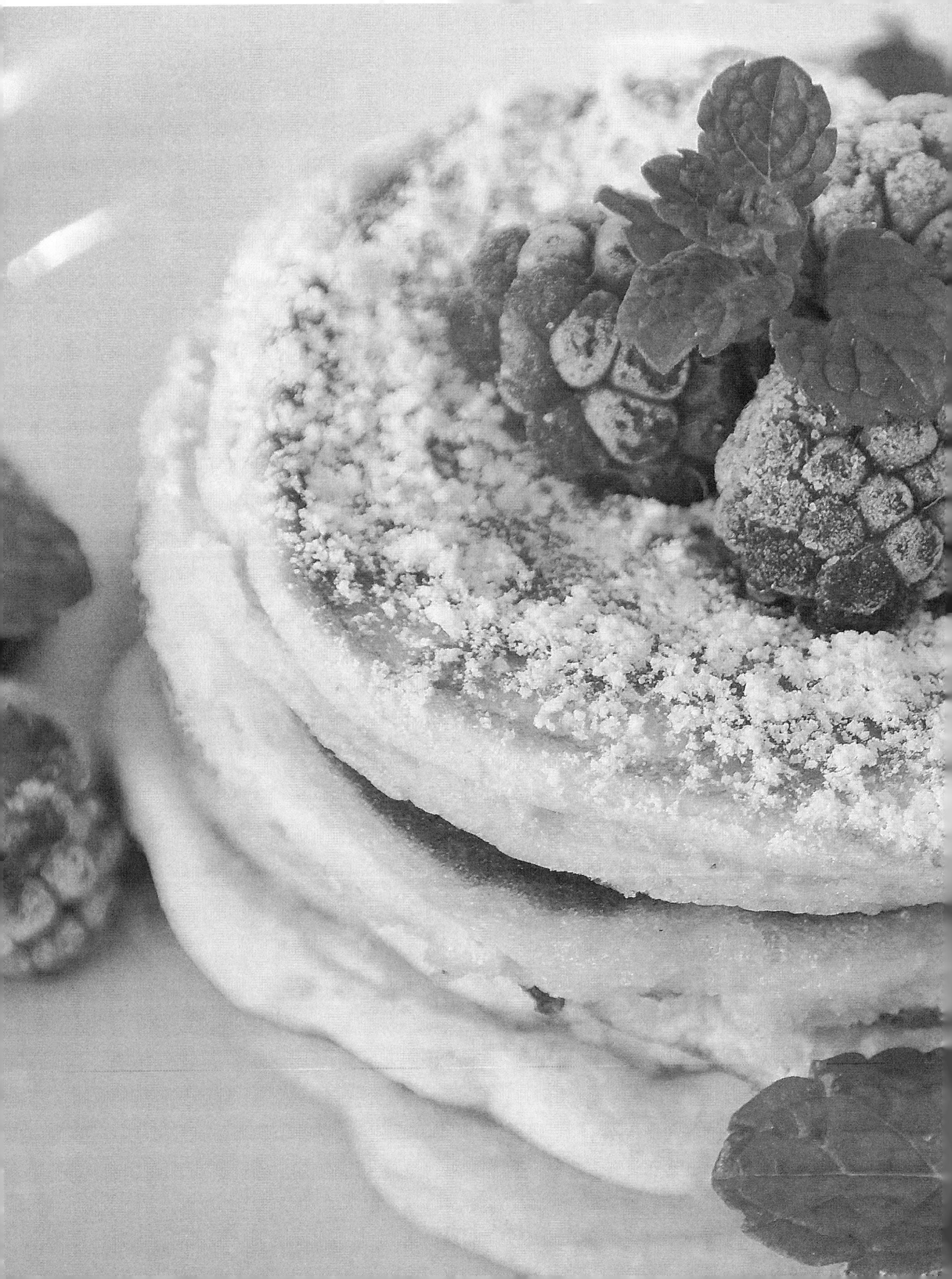

Sweet Treats

Chia Pudding `VEGAN` 174

Berry Crumble `VEGETARIAN` 175

Banana Birthday Cake with Lemon Icing `VEGETARIAN` 176

Brownie Cupcakes with Vanilla Icing `VEGETARIAN` 178

Rhubarb Custard Cup `VEGETARIAN` 180

Fluffy Pancakes `VEGETARIAN` 181

Chocolate Fudge Sauce `VEGAN` 182

Chocolate Raspberry Dessert `VEGETARIAN` 183

Christmas Mince Pie `VEGETARIAN` 184

Strawberry Ice Cream `VEGAN` 186

Ginger Cookies `VEGAN` 187

PB&J Mug Cake `VEGETARIAN` 188

Lemon Bar `VEGETARIAN` 189

Chia Pudding

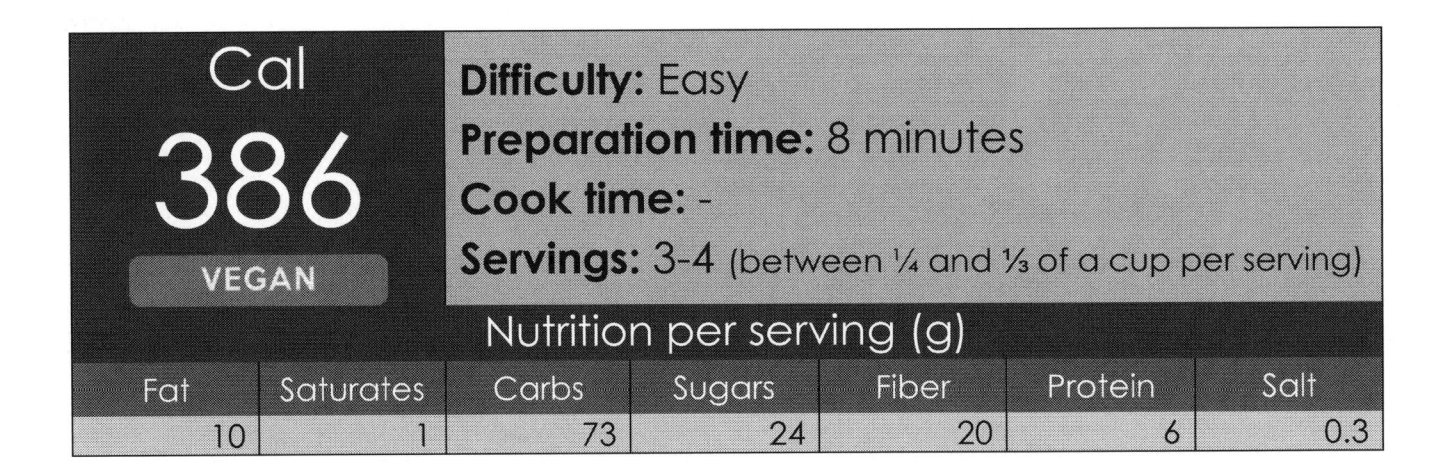

Cal 386 VEGAN

Difficulty: Easy
Preparation time: 8 minutes
Cook time: -
Servings: 3-4 (between ¼ and ⅓ of a cup per serving)

Nutrition per serving (g)

Fat	Saturates	Carbs	Sugars	Fiber	Protein	Salt
10	1	73	24	20	6	0.3

Ingredients

- ¼ cup chia seeds
- 1 tbsp cocoa powder
- 1 tbsp peanut butter
- 1 tbsp maple syrup
- 1 can coconut milk

Method

1. Fill an airtight jar with all the ingredients.

2. Close the jar and shake, then remove the top and stir the ingredients. Ensure that the bottom of the jar is clear. Shake again and place in the fridge for a minimum of 4 hours.

Berry Crumble

Cal 425
VEGETARIAN

Difficulty: Easy
Preparation time: 15 minutes
Cook time: 20 minutes
Servings: 3

Nutrition per serving (g)

Fat	Saturates	Carbs	Sugars	Fiber	Protein	Salt
22.2	5.7	52.2	22.6	3.6	5.7	0.3

Ingredients

Filling

- 1 cup blueberries, fresh or frozen
- 2 tbsp water
- 1 cup strawberries, fresh or frozen
- 1 ½ tsp white sugar
- 1 tbsp cornstarch, corn-based

Crumble

- 1 cup gluten-free cornflakes
- ¼ cup packed brown sugar
- ¼ cup gluten-free flour
- 3 tbsp dried coconut, shredded
- 2 tbsp pumpkin seeds
- 4 tbsp butter, softened

Method

1. Preheat the oven to 350°F.

2. In a bowl, crush the cornflakes into small bits and mix them with the brown sugar, flour, coconut, and pumpkin seeds. Use the softened butter to work the dry mix into small crumbs, making sure there are no large lumps.

3. In an ovenproof dish, place the strawberries and blueberries, cutting the strawberries into smaller pieces if necessary. Over the berries, sprinkle the white sugar and cornstarch. Spread the crumble over the top evenly. Place the dish on a flat baking tray and cook in the oven for 20 minutes. The topping should be golden brown.

4. It is best served hot.

Banana Birthday Cake with Lemon Icing

Cal 405 — VEGETARIAN

Difficulty: Medium
Preparation time: 15 minutes
Cook time: 55 minutes
Servings: 16

Nutrition per serving (g)

Fat	Saturates	Carbs	Sugars	Fiber	Protein	Salt
18	2.8	56.8	31	1.1	3.7	0.4

Ingredients

Cake
- ½ cup white sugar
- ½ cup brown sugar
- 1 cup butter, softened
- 3 eggs, large
- 2 tsp vanilla extract
- 4 bananas, firm, mashed
- 1 tsp chia seeds, can be substituted with 1 ½ tsp guar gum
- 1 tbsp boiling water
- 2 tsp of baking soda
- ½ cup lactose-free milk
- 3 cups gluten-free flour
- 2 tsp of baking powder

Icing
- 1 ½ tbsp lemon juice
- 5 tbsp butter
- 1 ½ cups powdered sugar
- 1 tbsp lemon zest

Method

1. Preheat the oven to 350°F. Grease a 10-inch round tin and line it with parchment paper.

2. In a bowl, mix the softened butter and sugar with a hand mixer until smooth and fluffy.

3. Add the vanilla and the eggs, one at a time.

4. Mash the bananas until there are 2 cups worth. Zest and juice the lemon and place the zest to the side. Add the banana and juice to the wet mix.

5. Dissolve the chia seeds in 1 tbsp of boiling water. Stir until the consistency is thick and then add to the wet mixture.

6   Heat the milk in the microwave for 30 seconds, then mix the baking soda into it. Fold into the wet mixture.

7   Sift together the flour and baking powder. Mix the dry ingredients into the wet mixture and stir until fully mixed. Pour into the cake tin and bake in the center of the oven for 45-60 minutes. When the cake turns golden, check the middle of the cake with a skewer to see if it is cooked. Remove it from the oven and allow to cool.

8   For the icing, pour the powdered sugar into a bowl. Soften the butter, but do not melt it. Add the dairy into the bowl. Begin mixing and add the lemon juice. Mix until smooth.

9   Ice the cake once it is cool and top with the lemon zest.

Brownie Cupcakes with Vanilla Icing

Cal 365
VEGETARIAN

Difficulty: Medium
Preparation time: 1 hour
Cook time: 20 minutes
Servings: 12

Nutrition per serving (g)

Fat	Saturates	Carbs	Sugars	Fiber	Protein	Salt
19.9	4.7	43.9	30.8	1.7	3.2	0.3

Ingredients

Cupcakes
- ½ cup butter
- 9 tbsp dark chocolate
- 2 eggs, large
- ¼ cup lactose-free milk
- 1 tsp vanilla extract
- 1 cup gluten-free flour
- 3 tbsp cocoa powder
- ¾ cup brown sugar
- ¼ tsp of baking powder
- ¾ tsp of baking soda
- Pinch of salt

Icing
- ½ cup butter
- 1 ½ cups powdered sugar
- ½ tsp vanilla extract
- 2 drops food coloring of choice
- Edible cake decorating pearls, optional

Method

1. Preheat the oven to 350°F. Line a muffin tray with cupcake liners.

2. Chop the chocolate roughly and melt it in the microwave with the butter for 15 seconds at a time, stirring in between.

3. Whisk the eggs, milk, and vanilla extract together until smooth, then add in the melted butter and chocolate.

4. In a separate bowl, mix the dry ingredients together then add in the wet mixture. Mix until the batter is smooth. Spoon an even amount of mixture into each cupcake liner.

5 Bake for 15 minutes, then check with a skewer. The top of the cupcakes should look slightly cracked and the skewer should come out clean. Remove the cupcakes from the oven and let the tin cool for 5 minutes before placing the cupcakes onto a cooling rack.

6 To make the icing, soften the butter, but don't melt it. Mix the butter, powdered sugar, vanilla extract, and 2 drops of food coloring in a bowl until it is smooth and creamy. If it is too dry, add a small amount of water. Ice the cupcakes once they are cool and decorate.

Rhubarb Custard Cup

Cal 431
VEGETARIAN

Difficulty: Easy
Preparation time: 5 minutes
Cook time: 20 minutes
Servings: 4

Nutrition per serving (g)

Fat	Saturates	Carbs	Sugars	Fiber	Protein	Salt
13.8	3.4	70.7	26.1	5	4.9	0.3

Ingredients

Rhubarb
- 1 ¼ cups rhubarb, fresh
- 2 ½ tbsp raspberries, fresh or frozen

Custard
- 4 tbsp custard powder, without milk or whey powder
- 4 cups lactose-free milk
- 1 ½ tbsp white sugar
- 1 tsp vanilla extract

Layer
- Low-FODMAP muesli or crumble

Method

1. Weigh and chop the rhubarb. Place the rhubarb and raspberries into a saucepan, cover with warm water, and place over medium heat and bring to a simmer. Allow to simmer for 10 minutes, then drain the liquid using a sieve. Mash the fruit in the saucepan.

2. In a microwave bowl, mix together the custard powder, milk, and white sugar. Cook on high for 2 minutes and stir, repeating until thick. Add vanilla extract if the flavor is not sweet enough.

3. Layer the rhubarb, custard, and muesli/crumble into cups.

Fluffy Pancakes

Cal 116 VEGETARIAN	**Difficulty:** Easy **Preparation time:** 10 minutes **Cook time:** 15 minutes **Servings:** 16 (4 per serving)

Nutrition per serving (g)

Fat	Saturates	Carbs	Sugars	Fiber	Protein	Salt
3.8	2	18.7	9.4	0.2	1.4	0.1

Ingredients

Batter
- 1 ¼ cups gluten-free flour
- 3 tsp baking powder
- 2 tbsp white sugar
- ¾ cup lactose-free or coconut milk
- 1 egg
- ¾ tsp vanilla extract
- 2 tsp butter

Serve
- ½ cup regular fat cream, whipped
- 8 tbsp strawberry jam

Method

1. In a bowl, whisk the dry ingredients and create a well in the middle. Add the milk, egg, and vanilla extract. Mix together until there are almost no lumps.

2. Test the batter. This is done by lifting the whisk out of the bowl. The batter should drizzle thickly back into the bowl; if it is too thick, add a tablespoon of milk.

3. Over medium heat, melt the butter in a non-stick pan. Wipe the pan with a paper towel to remove excess butter.

4. Place 2 tablespoons of batter per pancake into the pan. When bubbles appear on the top of the pancakes, flip them carefully and cook the other side until golden. Serve hot.

Chocolate Fudge Sauce

Cal 95
VEGAN

Difficulty: Easy
Preparation time: 5 minutes
Cook time: 20 minutes
Servings: 16 (1 ½ tbsp per serving)

Nutrition per serving (g)

Fat	Saturates	Carbs	Sugars	Fiber	Protein	Salt
5.4	4.4	12.3	10.4	0.7	0.6	0

Ingredients

- ⅔ cup coconut cream, canned
- 1 cup coconut milk, can substitute with other approved milk
- ¾ cup brown sugar
- 4 tbsp cocoa powder
- 3 tbsp coconut oil
- 1 tsp vanilla extract

Method

1. In a blender, mix the ingredients until smooth.

2. Transfer to a small saucepan over medium heat. Bring to a gentle boil for 20 minutes, stirring occasionally to stop the boiling and to mix in any skin that forms.

3. Place in the fridge to cool for 20 minutes. A thin skin will form; whisk it into the sauce. Overnight, the mixture will turn to a fudge-like consistency.

Chocolate Raspberry Dessert

Cal 280 VEGETARIAN	**Difficulty:** Easy **Preparation time:** 20 minutes **Cook time:** 15 minutes **Servings:** 12					

Nutrition per serving (g)

Fat	Saturates	Carbs	Sugars	Fiber	Protein	Salt
17	6.6	27	17.2	2.7	4.7	0.1

Ingredients

- 1 cup dark chocolate
- ½ cup butter
- ⅔ cup white sugar
- 4 eggs, large
- ½ cup gluten-free flour
- ½ tsp chia seeds, can be substituted with ½ tsp guar gum
- 2 tsp boiling water
- ¼ cup raspberries, fresh or frozen

Method

1. Preheat the oven to 400°F and line a muffin tray with 12 cupcake liners.

2. In a microwave bowl, break up the chocolate and microwave for 15 seconds. Stir and repeat heating for 10 seconds and stirring until melted.

3. Let the butter reach room temperature, then place it into a bowl with the sugar and whisk together until fluffy. Next, mix in the eggs, one at a time.

4. Soften the chia seeds in boiling water.

5. Beat in the flour and a pinch of salt until the mixture is smooth, then fold in the chocolate and chia seeds.

6. Spoon half the mixture into the cupcake liners and top with 1 or 2 raspberries, then cover with the remainder of the mixture.

7. Bake for 10-11 minutes, then remove when the top just starts to set. Cool for 10 minutes before removing from the tray.

Christmas Mince Pie

Cal 251 VEGETARIAN

Difficulty: Medium
Preparation time: 50 minutes
Cook time: 20 minutes
Servings: 12 (1 per serving)

Nutrition per serving (g)

Fat	Saturates	Carbs	Sugars	Fiber	Protein	Salt
11.1	1.8	33.9	14.3	1.3	4	0.1

Ingredients

Pastry
- 1 cup gluten-free flour
- ½ tsp guar gum
- 2 tbsp brown sugar
- ⅛ tsp cinnamon, ground
- ½ cup butter
- 1 tbsp lactose-free milk
- 1 egg, large

Fruit mince
- ⅔ cup rhubarb, fresh
- ⅓ cup imperial mandarin
- 3 ½ tbsp cranberries, dried
- 2 ½ tsp ginger, crystallized
- 3 tbsp brown sugar
- ¼ cup water
- ½ tsp allspice
- ½ tsp cloves, ground
- ½ tsp cinnamon, ground
- ¼ tsp ginger, ground
- ½ cup pumpkin seeds, toasted and chopped

Egg wash
- 1 egg
- 1 tbsp lactose-free milk

Method

1. Preheat the oven to 350°F. Grease a 12-hole shallow cupcake tin.

2. To make the pastry, sift the flour and guar gum into a large bowl, then stir the sugar and cinnamon in.

3. Chop the dairy into cubes and rub it into the flour until it looks like breadcrumbs.

4. In a bowl, heat the egg and mix it into the pastry with the milk. Bring the dough together and work it together until smooth. Pat the dough into a flat ball, wrap in plastic wrap, and chill in the fridge for 30 minutes.

5. For the fruit mince, start with the rhubarb by peeling and chopping it before roasting it in the preheated oven with a few tablespoons of water and brown sugar. After 10 minutes, the rhubarb should be soft.

6. Peel and chop the mandarin and crystallized ginger. Place a saucepan over medium heat. Add the fruit, water, and spices to the saucepan and bring it to a simmer. Once the rhubarb is cooked, add it to the saucepan and let it simmer for 10 minutes. Add more sugar and spices to taste, then mix in the pumpkin seeds.

7. Assemble the pie by first rolling the pastry out to ¼- inch thick and then cut the bases out to fit in the cupcake tin. Transfer the pastry to the tin and prick holes with a fork. Put 1 heaped spoon of fruit into each pie and top with strips of pastry.

8. Mix the egg and milk together, then brush that over the pastry and bake for 20 minutes.

Strawberry Ice Cream

Cal 177
VEGAN

Difficulty: Easy
Preparation time: 15 minutes
Cook time: -
Servings: 4

Nutrition per serving (g)

Fat	Saturates	Carbs	Sugars	Fiber	Protein	Salt
4	3.5	37	28.4	2.7	1.2	0.1

Ingredients

- 2 small bananas, firm and frozen
- 7 oz strawberries, frozen
- 5 tbsp coconut yogurt
- 2 tbsp maple syrup
- 1 tsp vanilla extract

Method

1 Chop the frozen fruit into small pieces, then place the ingredients into a food processor. Blend until smooth, making sure to scrape down the sides.

2 Taste the mixture and add maple syrup or vanilla extract as desired. Serve soft or freeze for a few hours before serving. Serve with chocolate fudge sauce.

Ginger Cookies

Cal 85
VEGAN

Difficulty: Easy
Preparation time: 10 minutes
Cook time: 20 minutes
Servings: 20-25 cookies (1-2 per serving)

Nutrition per serving (g)

Fat	Saturates	Carbs	Sugars	Fiber	Protein	Salt
3	1.5	13	1.8	1.8	2	0.1

Ingredients

- ½ cup warm water
- 2 tbsp chia seeds
- ½ cup brown sugar
- 2 tbsp coconut oil
- 3 tbsp ginger, ground
- 1 tbsp cinnamon
- 1 cup buckwheat flour
- 1 cup brown rice flour
- Peanut butter or dark chocolate for filling

Method

1. Preheat the oven to 350°F and line a baking tray with parchment paper.

2. Put the chia seeds into warm water and let sit for 5 minutes.

3. In a bowl, mix the chia seeds and water, sugar, oil, ginger, and cinnamon.

4. Add the flour slowly then create balls with the dough, 1 tablespoon per ball to start with. You can add more dough to make larger cookies. Place them on the baking tray.

5. Make a hole in each ball of dough before baking for 20 minutes.

6. Add the filling while the cookies are still warm.

PB&J Mug Cake

Cal 396 VEGETARIAN	Difficulty: Easy Preparation time: 2 minutes Cook time: 2 minutes Servings: 2

Nutrition per serving (g)

Fat	Saturates	Carbs	Sugars	Fiber	Protein	Salt
15.5	3.5	54.5	21	4	11.5	0.1

Ingredients

- 1 egg, large
- 3 tbsp almond milk
- 3 tbsp peanut butter
- 5 tbsp gluten-free flour
- 2 tbsp sugar
- 1 tbsp jam/jelly, preferred flavor

Method

1. In a large mug, mix the ingredients, except the jam/jelly.

2. Swirl the jam in the mug before cooking.

3. Microwave on high until the center is just cooked.

Lemon Bar

Cal 212
VEGETARIAN

Difficulty: Easy
Preparation time: 10 minutes
Cook time: 50 minutes
Servings: 16 (1-2 per serving)

Nutrition per serving (g)

Fat	Saturates	Carbs	Sugars	Fiber	Protein	Salt
7.3	5.2	35.1	25	1.4	3.4	0.1

Ingredients

Crust
- 1 ½ cups gluten-free flour
- ½ cup white sugar
- ½ cup butter, unsalted
- 2 tbsp water

Lemon
- 4 eggs, large
- ½ cup lemon juice
- 1 ½ cups sugar
- ¼ cup gluten-free flour
- Powdered sugar, to dust on top

Method

1. Preheat the oven to 350°F. Grease a square baking pan (9.5 inches by 9.5 inches) with butter and set aside.

2. Mix the flour and sugar together. Mix the butter into the flour until the mixture reaches a crumbly consistency. Add the water and mix well. Press into the bottom of the pan and bake for 20-25 minutes.

3. In another bowl, whisk the eggs, lemon juice, sugar, and flour until smooth. Pour onto the baked crust.

4. Bake for another 25 minutes, remove from the oven, and allow to cool.

Conclusion

With the high number of people around the world who struggle with digestive issues and the symptoms that go with them, there needs to be ways for them to cope. The low-FODMAP diet is aimed at people who have issues such as IBS, which is related to the way that food interacts with the digestive system. During the course of the diet, there are specific steps that are followed to aid in the control of symptoms.

The steps on the low-FODMAP diet aim at reducing the ingestion of high-FODMAPS to allow the body to reach a level of normalcy. Then there is the slow process of testing to see what foods cause the symptoms to flare up again. Throughout the course of this diet, each individual will discover how to create healthier eating habits. However, it must be remembered that this way of eating is not meant to be permanent as it can cause good bacteria that grow in our digestive system to stop being produced.

It is important to take all aspects of the diet into consideration. There are positives and negatives to any type of diet, and these need to be understood before starting the diet. The overall goal is to know and understand the different types of foods that can create symptoms when eaten. Use all the information accumulated through this guide and do your own research to set yourself up for a healthier lifestyle. Do not just rely on the diet to help with digestive symptoms; it is best to consult a healthcare professional such as a dietician to put together a full plan to combat the symptoms you are experiencing. A professional will also be able to guide you through the stages of the diet in a healthy way.

Remember to collect recipes whenever you can. Play around with the way you prepare food. Most of all, remember to stay the course. Diets are not easy; however, with perseverance, your life can be completely turned around.

Resources

The following is a list of resources that can be used to help with the low-FODMAP journey. There are a number of websites available to use; these can provide tips that help in the process of the diet.

Monash University:
As a university, they have put together a number of different resources for people to use. They ensure that there is new information uploaded and anything their team finds out is available to the public. They have an entire website built around the concept of a low-FODMAP diet. In addition to a website, Monash has also developed an app that you can use on your phone on a daily basis. This app aims to provide tools to help people with this diet. As a whole, Monash provides a lot of resources that can be used by anyone who is interested in the low-FODMAP diet. This is for people at all different stages of the diet, from beginner to someone who is trying to maintain their diet.
https://www.monashfodmap.com/

FODMAP Everyday Downloadable Resources
The FODMAP Everyday website was created to help individuals who are looking to use the low-FODMAP diet to relieve their IBS symptoms. As a whole, the site provides information about the diet, recipes, and articles. It is a user-friendly site that newcomers and veterans of the diet can use. It links to other sites, such as Monash, and provides resources that can be downloaded and used. There is also access to a shop where you can buy various items such as books, kitchen items, and food.
https://www.fodmapeveryday.com/

IBS Vegan
This website is specifically aimed at individuals who are vegan. The website caters to vegans who struggle with IBS. As well as information about IBS, they provide recipes that are vegan-friendly. This site is great for people who want to maintain their vegan lifestyle, while at the same time eating in a way that will help reduce their IBS symptoms.
http://www.ibsvegan.com/

Fody Foods
As a website, Fody mainly acts as an online store. Their focus is on selling low-FODMAP foods. This provides the opportunity for people struggling to find certain food items in stores to find what they want online. With shipping available, you do not have to be close to a store to buy their food items, which includes snacks, sauces, oils, and more. This is a great option for people who struggle to find time to make snacks and sauces.
https://www.fodyfoods.com/

There are many places to find resources on the Internet. There are a lot of websites with recipes and advice, and these will help with the maintenance of a low-FODMAP lifestyle. If you are unsure about using online resources, the best place to find help is with a professional. Dieticians and other healthcare professionals will be able to give you resources. The best option is to start working with a professional who can help you personalize an eating plan that will be best suited to you. They will also guide you in the right direction when it comes time to implement the different stages of the diet. There are also physical resources that are available. Books are a great place to discover information about food and new recipes.

References

Angelle, A. (2017, June 3). Irritable Bowel Syndrome: Symptoms, Treatment & Prevention. Retrieved from
https://www.livescience.com/34760-irritable-bowel-syndrome-diarrhea-constipation.htm

Chi, A. (2019). How does a Poor Diet Affect Your Digestive System? Retrieved from
https://www.livestrong.com/article/435030-how-does-a-poor-diet-affect-your-digestive-system/

IBS Diets. (2019, November 25). FODMAP Dieting Guide. Retrieved from
https://www.ibsdiets.org/fodmap-diet/fodmap-food-list/

Paul, R. (2017, January 4). The Top 5 Benefits of Switching to a Low-FODMAP Diet this Year; Free yourself from IBS. Retrieved from
https://www.rachelpaulsfood.com/top-5-benefits-switching-low-fodmap-diet-2017/

Stanford (2014, January). The Low FODMAP Diet (FODMAP= Fermentable Oligo-Di-Monosaccharides and Polyols). Retrieved from
http://www.marinhealthcare.org/upload/Low-FODMAP-Diet.pdf

Made in the USA
Monee, IL
21 April 2020